362.1
Som

JUN 2 4 2010

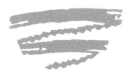

GETTING WHAT WE DESERVE

GETTING WHAT WE DESERVE

Health and
Medical Care
in AMERICA

Alfred Sommer, M.D., M.H.S.

Former Dean, Johns Hopkins
Bloomberg School of Public Health

THE JOHNS HOPKINS UNIVERSITY PRESS
Baltimore

© 2009 The Johns Hopkins University Press
All rights reserved. Published 2009
Printed in the United States of America on acid-free paper
9 8 7 6 5 4 3 2 1

The Johns Hopkins University Press
2715 North Charles Street
Baltimore, Maryland 21218-4363
www.press.jhu.edu

Library of Congress Cataloging-in-Publication Data
Sommer, Alfred, 1942–
   Getting what we deserve : health and medical care in America / Alfred Sommer.
    .p. ; cm.
   Includes bibliographical references and index.
   ISBN-13: 978-0-8018-9387-2 (hardcover : alk. paper)
   ISBN-10: 0-8018-9387-9 (hardcover : alk. paper)
1. Public health—United States. 2. Health. 3. Medical policy—United States. I. Title.
[DNLM: 1. Health Status—United States. 2. Health Policy—United States. 3. Public
Health—United States. 4. Social Medicine—United States. WA 300 AA1 S697h 2009]
   RA445.S66 2009
   362.1—dc22   2009006039

A catalog record for this book is available from the British Library.

Special discounts are available for bulk purchases of this book. For more information, please contact
Special Sales at 410-516-6936 or specialsales@press.jhu.edu.

The Johns Hopkins University Press uses environmentally friendly book materials, including
recycled text paper that is composed of at least 30 percent post-consumer waste, whenever
possible. All of our book papers are acid-free, and our jackets and covers are printed on
paper with recycled content.

To
　Jill, Charles, Marni, and Albert

To
　M. R. B.
　(who instantly got it!)

　and to my mentors, colleagues, and students
　who taught me to read the fine print—
　but never lose sight of the big picture

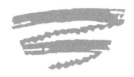

Contents

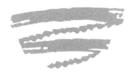

Preface

Let's not go through the thick of thin things.
—Arthur Jampolsky, 1999

This book presents a personal perspective about things that make a difference in the health of individuals and of populations. After forty years straddling the divide between clinical medicine and public health, I find that information on critical issues can be too confusing for most informed readers to grasp, while misinformation (purposeful and otherwise) interferes with personal choices and rational public debate. Particularly perplexing and discouraging is our society's continuing fascination with the biological causes of disease, when behavioral, societal, and economic factors play important roles. Hope (and hype) has been invested in the "genetic revolution," yet most major diseases would respond to changes in the environment in which our genes work, an environment frequently of our own choosing. Misinformation is often responsible for the divide between scientific evidence and the way medicine is practiced.

I have had the privilege of observing the medical enterprise from multiple perspectives. Early in my training, all that was important was mastering new drugs, tests, and procedures. I soon realized that Harvard Medical School's strongest asset was that it was not tethered to a single teaching hospital. Instead, we honed our clinical skills at bedsides in five or six major hospitals within Harvard's orbit. My most illuminating lesson was that, while none of these illustrious hospitals was more than a few miles from the others, their physicians often treated the same clinical condition in different ways. These differences were not because one hospital's clinicians were better than another's, but because traditions and cultures differed and available clinical evidence did not sufficiently support the value of one tradition over another. This observation encouraged my congenital cynicism regarding dogma in general and clinical dogma in particular.

After having spent a lifetime in a tiny specialty (ophthalmology) broadened immensely by a long and personal involvement in epidemiology and global health, I have realized that we must think about health and disease, and the ways we approach them, in radically different ways. Most premature deaths in the United States are caused by known and preventable factors; greater expenditures on basic research are not needed to solve these problems, nor are increases in health care spending.

The rest of the developed world spends a great deal less on health care than we do but lives healthier and longer lives. This paradox seems too complex to understand and too complicated to reverse because we have lost sight of the essentials—thanks in large part to the obfuscations of pharmaceutical marketing, the entrenched interests of the medical insurance industry, the political timidity and rigid philosophies of our politicians and business leaders, and sheer lack of imagination. This is all the more striking when other countries provide successful models that we could choose to emulate without fear of falling into an unknown abyss.

Ponder a few absurdities:

1. The United States spends nearly twice as much on health care as does the rest of the developed world but has higher infant mortality and shorter longevity than most developed nations.

2. We have a plethora of drugs of widely varying costs that accomplish the same end—and nearly all are cheaper when acquired abroad.

3. Our average life span nearly doubled over the past century, before we discovered effective drugs for most diseases or even thought about ways to change our genome.

4. Almost all newly developed treatments are expensive, but their benefits are generally marginal.

This slim volume recounts verities, ironies, and inconsistencies at the core of what we have been led to believe is an insolvably complex problem. What I hope to make clear is that the core issues are not all complex, nor are they insolvable. To act appropriately, we simply need to understand their essence.

If I am accused of oversimplifying, I hope it is for exposing the essence of an issue and not for ignoring nuances at the margins.

I thank the Johns Hopkins University for the opportunity to serve as the dean of its Bloomberg School of Public Health. Its faculty introduced me to concepts and domains I'd never known existed, its students stimulated me to think and act across the artificial boundaries and narrow perspectives that separate "medicine" from "public health," and its supporters challenged me to convey my synthesis and insights to a larger audience.

I also thank those who assisted me in the preparation of this manuscript: Rebecca Pickard, my assistant; Meg Thompson, who offered useful editorial suggestions; and Wendy Harris and Linda Forlifer of the Johns Hopkins University Press, for their editing skills and for shepherding this book to publication.

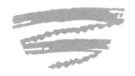

GETTING WHAT WE DESERVE

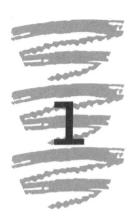

GENESIS

From Few to Many—in Fits and Starts

Populations grow when the number of children who are born and survive exceeds the number of people who die. For most of human history, life was "nasty, brutish, and short," and life and death were exquisitely balanced. More than a few women never survived labor; fewer children survived infancy. But enough survived to establish viable extended families, which occasionally grew large enough to form clans, tribes, and eventually nations. Nothing very large, mind you, until the increased productivity associated with the domestication of agriculture allowed for large, settled communities and the "excess" labor (and food) could be diverted to the construction of great monuments, art, and the year-round staffing of armies. This productivity led to the first great population explosion. Then, for an inordinately long period, the world stopped growing.

Population expansion led to cities, and urban development came with crowding, filth, and the ready spread of communicable diseases. Wars and plague periodically depopulated the countryside;

World Population

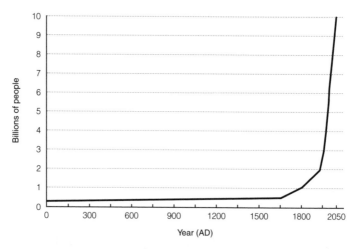

FIGURE 1. THE POPULATION WAS FLAT.
Estimates of the world's population from 1 CE to 2050. For nearly two thousand years, the population of the globe remained largely unchanged, at fewer than half a billion people. The number of people on the planet began its dizzying ascent only in the 1700s. Source: Data from a series of publications of the United Nations and the U.S. Census Bureau, assuming medium global fertility rates beyond the year 2000.

without the agricultural production of the countryside, cities starved.

In the fourteenth century, the Black Death (plague), spread to humans by infected fleas jumping from dying rats, wiped out one-third of Europe's population, more than 25 million people.[1] Asia was hit even harder. Whole societies collapsed in fear, famine, and chaos. Fields were abandoned, commerce ceased, cities emptied, and superstition and persecution reigned. Medieval districts of many European cities sport elaborately wrought "plague pillars," fanciful monuments erected by the survivors in thanks for God's intercession. China's population experienced recurrent cycles of expansion followed by implosion as feast alternated with famine, accompanied by the diseases and political instability with which poor harvests and famine are frequently linked.

For millennia, the world's population did not change, give or take a few hundred million (Figure 1). Between 8000 BCE and 1750 CE, the world's population doubled every twenty-five hundred years. Since 1945, the world's population has been doubling every thirty-six years.

Population expansion largely reflects increased chances that children will survive their earliest years of life. C. P. Snow observed

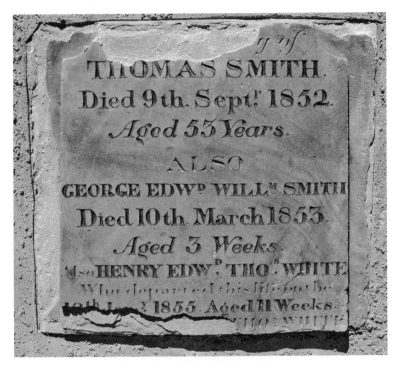

FIGURE 2. UNTIL RECENTLY, PEOPLE DIED YOUNG.
A tombstone in St. David's Park, a former cemetery in Hobart, Australia, records one death at age 53 and two deaths before the fourth month of life. For most of human history, life expectancy (from birth) was short, which is why populations barely grew. Source: Photo by Alfred Sommer.

that, "in eighteenth century French villages, the median age of marriage was older than the median age of death."[2] More than half of all people died before they were old enough to marry—indeed, much before! During the Middle Ages, half the children in Western societies died before the age of 5. The average age of death—traditionally defined as average life expectancy at birth—was 5 years (or less). The average age of marriage was the late teens, 10 to 15 years older.

Gravestones in a park overlooking Hobart, Australia (but they could be in a cemetery nearly anywhere in the world), graphically tell the tale. One gravestone reads much like the others: Thomas Smith, died 1852, aged 53 years; George Edward William Smith, died 1853, aged 3 weeks; Henry Edward Thomas White, died 1855, aged 11 weeks (Figure 2). Many infants (and mothers) succumbed to the rigors of childbirth or to the privations—infection, exposure, and malnutrition—that followed.

Much had changed by the dawn of the twentieth century. The median age of death in England and Wales had risen to 33 years, well beyond the median age of marriage. Still, nearly a third of all those who died were younger than 5. By 1966, the median age of death was 73, and nearly half of all those who died were older than 75 (Figure 3).

The capacity of people to envision so dramatic a change was constricted by life's experiences. Rousseau proclaimed that "50 percent of children die by the age of 8 and always will—it's natural law."[3] By the early years of the twentieth century, Rousseau's eighteenth-century natural law had been completely rewritten. It is still being rewritten.

In most societies, even in poor Asian countries such as Bangladesh, population growth has begun once again to slow. This is not because large numbers of children are dying—precisely the opposite. With the likelihood of children's survival vastly increased,

Age of Death – England and Wales

1891

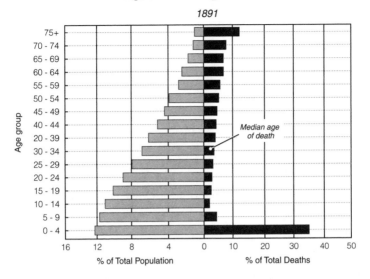

1966

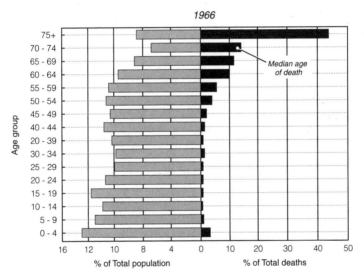

FIGURE 3. AGE OF DEATH IN ENGLAND AND WALES (1891 AND 1966).
In 1891, the median age of death was 33 years (roughly half of those who died were younger, and half were older). More than one-third of all deaths were children under 5 years of age. By 1966, seventy years later, the median age of death was 73 years, forty years older than it had been in 1891. Only 3 percent of deaths were children under 5 years of age, while nearly half who died were over age 75.
Source: Adapted, with permission, from World Development Report (Oxford: Oxford University Press, 1993), 31, Box Figure 1.4.

women no longer need to give birth to four to eight infants just to ensure that one or two male offspring will survive to provide for their old age. Family-planning services have given women a choice, and as they have gained education and independence, they have opted for, as one wag put it, "investing in fewer, high-quality children, instead of counting on the lottery of large numbers." As retirement funds have taken over financial responsibility for elderly people, urban dwellings have become less spacious, and raising and educating children have become vastly more expensive, fertility rates in some wealthy countries (Italy, Spain, Japan) have fallen below "replacement" levels.

Why did life expectancy suddenly, and dramatically, begin to increase? Because the number of young people who died declined dramatically. Death at 1 year of age lowers overall life expectancy a lot more than does death at 67. Life expectancy has dramatically increased because the young survive, not because the elderly live longer!

More of the young survive because living conditions have dramatically improved. Between 1900 and 1950, years before development of the first measles vaccine, measles deaths in the United States declined by more than 95 percent (Figure 4). Tuberculosis deaths in the United States declined by 90 percent over roughly the same period—long before there was a drug with which to effectively treat the disease (Figure 5).

The risks of early childhood infections fell because children (and those who cared for them) lived in more hygienic, more sanitary environments with better-ventilated homes, schools, and workplaces. Because they were also better fed, they were more resistant to the serious complications of the infections they contracted. Plenty of children and young adults still died of infectious diseases, but not as often.

Hippocrates recognized the importance that living conditions had on health. In "Airs, Waters and Places," he advised itinerant physicians that, to best care for patients, they should understand the environment in which they lived. He did not know anything about microbial agents, but he recognized that slovenly environments bred disease. Social and medical reformers of the late nineteenth century, such as Rudolph Virchow, predicted that dramatic improvements in health depended foremost on improving living conditions—particularly those of the poor. In general, everyone suffered from the traditional "curse of the commons": the wealthy could modestly improve the environment immediately around them but

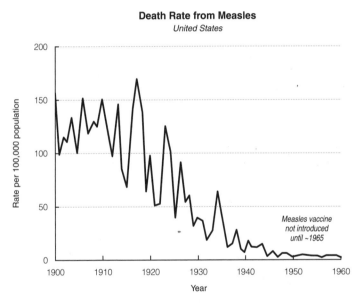

Death Rate from Measles
United States

FIGURE 4. BETTER NUTRITION AND PUBLIC HEALTH MEASURES MATTER. Death rates from measles in the United States, 1900–1960. Between 1900 and 1960, annual measles death rates declined by more than 95 percent, long before the introduction of an effective measles vaccine. Although the number of measles cases remained high, children were better nourished, housed, and clothed and therefore were less likely to suffer from severe, life-threatening complications of their infection. Source: Data from the Centers for Disease Control and Prevention, *Vital Statistics of the United States* (www.cdc.gov/nchs/products/pubs/pubd/vsus/vsus.htm).

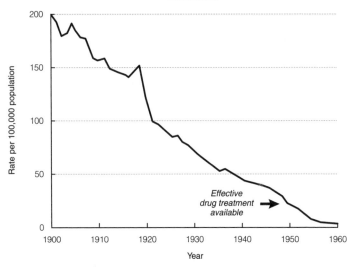

Death Rate from Tuberculosis
United States

FIGURE 5. BETTER NUTRITION AND PUBLIC HEALTH MEASURES MATTER.
Death rates from tuberculosis in the United States, 1900–1960. Deaths from tuberculosis declined steadily long before there was an effective drug for treating the
disease. Public health measures (case finding, sanitation, and more effective quarantine) and better housing reduced the rate of transmission of tuberculosis.
Better-nourished and healthier individuals were more resistant to infection by the
tubercle bacillus and to its complications. Source: Data from the Centers for Disease
Control and Prevention, *Vital Statistics of the United States* (www.cdc.gov/nchs/products/
pubs/pubd/vsus/vsus.htm).

failed to invest in the massively defiled environments of the poor—
environments that fostered the spread of disease that ultimately
entrapped everyone, rich and poor alike.

Recognition and acceptance of new medical insights, particularly
the ways in which infections spread, played a major role in advancing health during the nineteenth century. Unfortunately, putting
these new ideas into medical practice badly lagged behind their
discovery. The young Hungarian physician Ignaz Semmelweis recognized that women giving birth in Vienna General Hospital's First

Obstetrical Clinic had two different experiences: women assisted by nurses (who routinely scrubbed their hands between deliveries and dressed in starched, immaculate uniforms) fared much better than did women assisted by physicians and medical students (who often came straight from the autopsy room covered in the blood and gore of the deceased and who almost never bothered to wash before delivering an infant).

Like so many medical reformers before and since, Semmelweis was vilified for daring to question the established medical paradigm. He was expelled from his academic position and died in an insane asylum at age 47. More on "evidence-based medicine" later.

The moral of the story: dramatic improvements in life expectancy in the United States and the rest of the Western world over the past 150 years have had a great deal more to do with improvements in standards of living and basic public health measures than with the discovery of new drugs and other therapeutic interventions (as important as those might be to the individuals who needed them). McKinlay and McKinlay estimate that, between 1900 and 1970, only 3.5 percent of the decline in total mortality, at most, could be "ascribed to medical measures."[4]

How could that be?

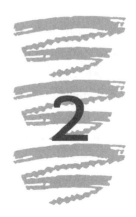

Disease Is the Sum
of All Evils

We've come to think of disease as an abnormal condition caused by a single, specific biological agent, such as a microbe or a mutated gene. Many such singular biological agents have been discovered. But health is not merely the absence of disease, nor do the origins of disease lie solely in the biological sphere. Julio Frenk (Mexico's recent Minister of Health) and others keep reminding us that health and disease result from the interplay of biological, social, economic, and cultural factors. Bugs and genes are important, but so is behavior—what we do to ourselves—and how we relate to our environment and to other people—what we do to them and what they do to us. This totality is far more complex and difficult to disentangle than is the role of isolated biological agents, but it also offers vastly expanded opportunities for advancing health, individually and collectively.

The collapse of Russian society that followed the breakup of the Soviet Union provides a frighteningly recent example of what can happen when the complex underpinnings of health are disrupted: between 1990 and 1993 (over three short years), Russian men lost five years of life expectancy! This calamity had many "fathers": a degraded public health system allowed preventable diseases to flourish (the rate of typhoid fever increased threefold; diphtheria and measles, fourfold); vaccines and medical supplies vanished from the marketplace; and economic despair and social isolation caused many men to literally drink themselves to death. The health of Russian women deteriorated as well, but not to the same extent.

INFECTION

The first among the biological factors—perhaps because we know more and can do more about it—is infection.

In 1969, U.S. Surgeon General William H. Stewart allegedly told Congress that it was "time to close the books on infectious disease." And so it might have seemed. Childhood infections, once the great killers of Western children, had been largely contained. Potable water and more sanitary living conditions had dramatically reduced the risks of diarrhea, typhoid, and typhus. Measles, diphtheria, smallpox, polio, and tetanus were prevented by vaccines. Postpartum infection ("puerperal sepsis"), the cause of many maternal deaths, had dramatically declined with the introduction of cleaner delivery techniques. Pneumonia and other bacterial infections responded rapidly to antibiotics. Unfortunately, in his optimism Stewart had overlooked the tenacity of microbes: high rates of mutation and reproduction ensured their ability to adapt to antibiotics and even to some potential vaccines, evolving in ways that improved their own survival.

Microbes have a relatively simple relationship with their host: if the host dies, the microbe dies (unless one of its offspring first hitches a ride on another host). A microbe that is both highly contagious and highly lethal will kill off many of its potential human hosts (as happened during the Black Death of the Middle Ages and the influenza pandemic of 1918–19).

Occasionally, human pathogens have killed off virtually every human host within a limited geographic range. This was obviously bad for both the host and the pathogen. More often, some humans (and the causative pathogen) survive. In ways that we do not yet fully understand, offspring of the surviving humans and the surviving pathogens became better able to co-exist. When measles was first introduced into the Faro Islands, a large proportion of the native population died. Subsequent epidemics were far more attenuated and less lethal. Smallpox, introduced into the Americas by European explorers and traders, wiped out much of the native population. Some estimate that, by the time the Pilgrims arrived, the native population of New England had been reduced to 10 percent of its previous level. But the rest of the population survived, and their offspring were far less likely to die from the disease.

Four thousand years ago, this delicate balance of mutually assured destruction between microbial pathogens and their human hosts had replaced food as the factor limiting population growth. By the dawn of the twentieth century, better sanitation, hygiene, housing, and nutrition had dramatically altered the equation. Antibiotics, which came into widespread use after World War II, changed the situation even more, but not as completely or as lastingly as Stewart and colleagues had thought.

Antibiotics were fantastically effective when they were first introduced, but even then, they rarely destroyed all of the harmful microbes they encountered. A few hardy pathogens, slightly altered by mutations in their genetic code, survived and reproduced. When again challenged by the same antibiotic, more survived than had the last time; those that evolved the greatest resistance to the antibiotic survived the most (and developed an efficient means for sharing their genetically evolved antibiotic resistance with their neighbors). Each time a host was infected and the patient was treated with the same antibiotic, the most resistant pathogens were "selected" for survival. This cycle, repeated innumerable times for many combinations of microbes and the antibiotics used to kill them, has given rise, over less than half a century, to a distressingly large number of highly resistant, deadly pathogens, such as methicillin-resistant Staphylococcus aureus (MRSA), vancomycin-resistant enterococcus (VRE), and extensively drug-resistant tuberculosis (XDR-TB).[1] This is a war without end. The slow, inexorable survival of the mutated fittest among microbial pathogens means that the conflict will never be won—at least, not by us!

Unfortunately, the pipeline of new antimicrobial drugs has shrunk dramatically. Pharmaceutical firms have chosen to invest instead in the discovery of "blockbuster" drugs for treating chronic conditions, drugs that large numbers of people will choose to use for the rest of their lives. The discovery of new antimicrobials needs fresh incentives if we are to keep up our side of this armaments race.

SMALLPOX

Pathogens can be immensely instructive. Smallpox exemplifies conditions under which we can vanquish a dreaded disease. Polio and HIV/AIDS are microbes that have successfully exploited human behavior to fight another day. SARS, like other "new" diseases menacing humans, emerged from nowhere to become a global threat. Human papilloma virus (HPV), Helicobacter pylori, and other microbes are now known to be responsible for diseases that until recently were thought to be of nonmicrobial origin.

Smallpox stands (to date) as the only naturally occurring disease, infectious or otherwise, eradicated from the face of the earth (that it still survives in laboratories is a cause for concern, but beyond this discussion). Why were we able to eradicate smallpox, which had probably killed tens of millions of people over millennia? The question one might more profitably and provocatively ask is, "Why did it take so long?"

As every schoolchild knows (or should), Jenner discovered the first vaccine in 1796, when he noted that milkmaids, commonly infected with cowpox, rarely came down with smallpox. He saved James Phipps's life by inoculating him with serum taken from a milkmaid's cowpox pustule—more or less the same "vaccine" that was used, nearly two hundred years later, to eradicate the disease.

As it turns out, smallpox was unique among globally infectious threats: there were no unapparent infections (anyone sick enough to infect others was covered by a nasty-looking rash, pustules, or scabs); there was no animal reservoir (the virus that caused human disease lived only in humans); there was a long incubation period (the time between first being infected and then becoming ill and infectious); and vaccination during the first third of the incubation period prevented clinical disease and any chance of infecting others.

Smallpox was finally eradicated when the World Health Assembly provided sufficient commitment and resources to vaccinate as many people as was practicable and, even more important, employed ongoing research to devise and deploy better tools for blocking the transmission of the virus from an infected person to a healthy person. These included a freeze-dried, stable vaccine; the bifurcated needle that required far less vaccine—effectively quintupling vaccine supplies when they were in shortest supply (Figure 6); and field procedures that focused available resources on vaccinating people who were likely to infect others—those individuals who had been in contact with active cases of disease and therefore at risk of having become infected themselves (Figure 7).[2]

In the end, the deed was done! In 1967 there had been 2.7 million smallpox deaths and the disease was endemic in thirty-one countries. The last naturally occurring case of smallpox was identified less than a decade later, in 1976. After a "waiting period" to ensure

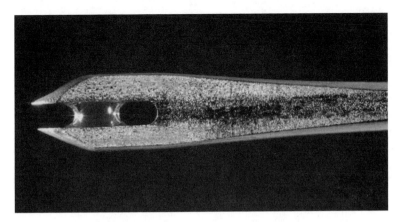

FIGURE 6. THE WORKING END OF THE BIFURCATED NEEDLE.
During the 1960s, a special needle was developed for administering smallpox vaccine. It captured a tiny amount of vaccine between its two prongs, and this amount proved to be as effective as the much larger drop of vaccine used in previous procedures. This effectively quintupled smallpox vaccine supplies at a time when stockpiles were inadequate to meet global needs. Source: Photo from the Centers for Disease Control and Prevention.

that eradication was indeed complete, the world was declared smallpox-free in 1980. Not a moment too soon! As we now know, the first AIDS cases were diagnosed the following year. HIV/AIDS drastically interferes with the immune response, a response critical to inducing immunity against future smallpox and to protecting the person vaccinated from complications associated with uncontrolled replication of the vaccine's own live virus. Once HIV/AIDS was loose in a population, widespread vaccination with the current vaccine would have been unthinkable, and eradication would have been impossible.

Carpe diem!

POLIO
Polio was the next viral disease targeted for eradication. While this has not yet happened, many of us remain hopeful that it soon

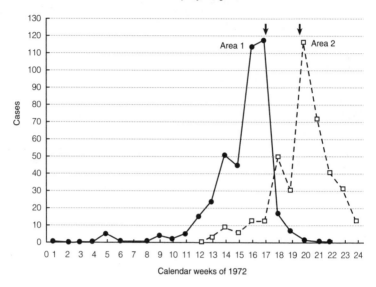

Smallpox Outbreaks
Khulna Municipality, Bangladesh - 1972

FIGURE 7. "RING VACCINATION" REALLY WORKS.

The effects of "surveillance and containment" (now called "ring vaccination") on the smallpox epidemic in Khulna Municipality, Bangladesh, 1972. Soon after the initiation of control activities (identification of all active cases of smallpox and vaccination of their contacts), indicated by the arrows, the number of new smallpox cases in the two neighborhoods declined rapidly. The brief lag between the start of control activities and the fall in new cases of clinical disease reflects the time it took to locate cases and vaccinate their contacts, the incubation period between infection with the smallpox virus and the onset of clinical disease, and the delay between vaccination and the onset of the protection it provided (vaccination prevented clinical smallpox among individuals vaccinated as late as five days after their initial infection with the virus). The incubation period (the time between exposure to the virus and the onset of clinical smallpox among nonvaccinated individuals) was twelve to fourteen days. Source: Adapted, with permission, from A. Sommer and S. Foster, "The 1972 Smallpox Outbreak in Khulna Municipality, Bangladesh. I. Methodology and Epidemiologic Findings," *American Journal of Epidemiology* 99 (1974): 294, Figure 1.

will. The eradication of polio poses significantly more challenges than did the eradication of smallpox: most people infected by the polio virus suffer nothing more than a mild, flulike illness. Therefore, most of those who are capable of transmitting the disease to others remain unknown. The vaccine itself is a good deal more complicated, as the live form of the vaccine is shed in the stool and can, occasionally, cause paralytic polio among those who come in contact with it and become infected. Finally, several strains of polio need to be included within the vaccine.

Despite these complexities, polio has, rather remarkably, been eradicated from much of the world, including Europe, the Americas, and the Western Pacific. Between 1988 and 2000, the annual number of polio cases worldwide dropped from 350,000 to 719. This was accomplished through careful surveillance for cases, identification of responsible strains, and universal childhood immunization. Between 1988 and 2005, an estimated 5 million children were saved from disabling paralysis, and 1.5 million deaths were averted (Figure 8).

While it is impossible to immunize everyone, enough children were immunized to dramatically reduce the risks of polio in virtually every part of the world. Until, that is, the fundamentalist governor of Kano State, Nigeria, refused to allow immunization, claiming that it was a Western plot against Islam. From Kano State, polio spread to twelve neighboring African countries from which it had already been eradicated and, via pilgrims congregating in Mecca for the Haj, far beyond. While Kano's governor has much to answer for, we should remember that vaccine-preventable outbreaks still occur in the United States, in communities that refuse to vaccinate their children for religious or other reasons (the well-educated, upscale community on Vashon Island, off the coast of Seattle—where 18 percent of children are unvaccinated—comes immediately to mind). Vociferous parent groups in the United States and Europe now

Polio Eradication Progress
1988

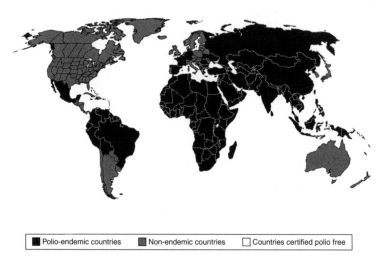

| ■ Polio-endemic countries | ■ Non-endemic countries | □ Countries certified polio free |

Polio Eradication Progress
1994

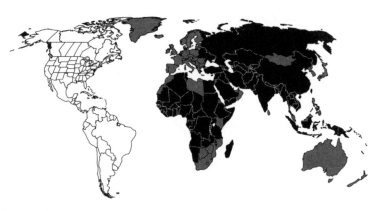

FIGURE 8. POLIO ERADICATION: DRAMATIC RESULTS—AND A NEAR MISS.
Global polio status, 1988–2003. The number of countries with endemic, wild-strain polio has shrunk dramatically since the onset of global polio eradication efforts.

blame vaccines for autism, diabetes, and a host of other ills, despite the absence of serious scientific evidence to support these claims. The absence of evidence has not dulled the ferocity of their beliefs or their advocacy. It has, however, confused other parents, created

Polio Eradication Progress
1998

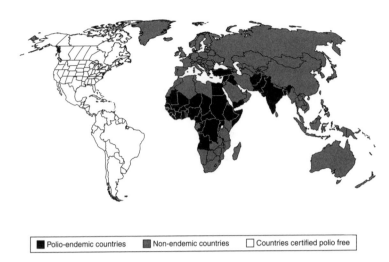

■ Polio-endemic countries   ■ Non-endemic countries   □ Countries certified polio free

Polio Eradication Progress
2003

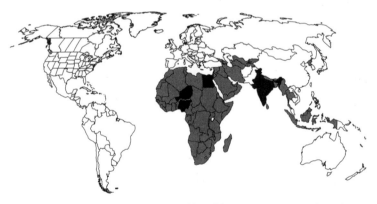

Source: Reprinted by permission from the World Health Organization (www.who.int/
features/2004/polio/en/#).

---

opposition to universal immunization, and raised the risk of real infections, and epidemics, in their communities.[3]

Nigeria has since changed its stance, and the world has redoubled its efforts to eradicate polio, as have the three other major

Countries Reporting Cases of Wild Poliovirus Infection in 2006 and Routes of Viral Spread from Countries with Endemic Disease from 2002 to 2006

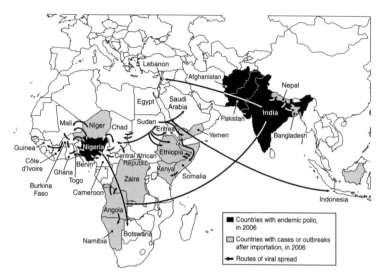

FIGURE 9. PERSISTENT CLUSTERS POSE CONTINUING RISKS.
Polio-endemic countries and the spread of infection, 2006. By 2006, only four countries still harbored the endemic spread of polio. One country in particular, Nigeria, was responsible for the importation of polio into twelve neighboring countries from which it had already been eradicated. Source: Reprinted by permission from M. Pallansch and H. S. Sandhu, "Eradication of Polio: Progress and Challenges," *New England Journal of Medicine* 355 (2006): 2509. Copyright © 2006 Massachusetts Medical Society. All rights reserved.

countries with ongoing transmission: India, Pakistan, and Afghanistan (Figure 9). It takes more than a village; it takes a globe!

HIV/AIDS, SARS, AVIAN FLU, AND OTHER VIRUSES THAT RECENTLY JUMPED THE SPECIES BARRIER

We've battled (and suffered from) the polio and smallpox viruses for millennia. HIV (human immunodeficiency virus), the cause of AIDS, was discovered only a few decades ago.[4] It is already our generation's "black death." Whole societies of sub-Saharan Africa have been decimated by the disease, which has left a trail of orphans, abandoned fields, and political instability and poverty in its wake. More than 10 million people have died of the disease, more than 30 million live with the infection (most won't live for long because they are poor people with little access to life-extending therapy—though recent international efforts and local initiatives have begun to treat growing numbers), and nearly 3 million become newly infected each year.

We know precisely how HIV is transmitted: like syphilis before it, through contact of the most intimate sort (primarily sex and the sharing of contaminated needles). Most sexual transmission of HIV would never occur if people simply used condoms. But with notable exceptions (Thailand, Uganda), sexual behavior has proved hard to change (see Chapter 5). It is particularly difficult for young women in traditional societies, especially sub-Saharan Africa, to "negotiate" safe sex. In Thailand and elsewhere, many faithful, married women are becoming infected by philandering husbands. Immunization would prove easier, but all the usual approaches (and some new and innovative ones) to vaccine development have failed to induce meaningful resistance against this elusive virus; it keeps changing its immune profile while directly attacking our bodies' immunological defenses.

HIV is just one example of the continuous emergence of new viral agents that, seeking new hosts, eventually assault humans. Most adopt to other animal species first, where they continue to multiply, mutate, and evolve, ultimately gaining the ability to "jump" from their animal reservoir to humans (not because of any malignant intent—it's just the way evolution and natural selection work).

SARS (severe acute respiratory syndrome) was one such virus, a potentially devastating "bullet" that we thankfully dodged! How? By rigorously applying basic public health principles: identify and isolate all cases and contacts. This broke the chain of transmission, but only because SARS was not particularly contagious. With rare exception, those sufficiently ill to transmit the virus required hospitalization, which is why most transmission occurred in hospitals and most of those infected were health care workers. Had the virus that caused SARS been more infectious, like seasonal flu, it could have circled the world, caused a global pandemic, and completely outstripped our capacity for control. Both the human host and the original animal-adapted virus (wherever it remains in hiding) have survived to fight another day.

The recent panic (and remaining concerns) over avian flu is built on several premises: there will be a deadly flu pandemic, perhaps even worse than the global "Spanish flu" pandemic of 1918–19 that may have killed as many as 40 million people, because, historically, "one is due"; the virus will be highly contagious, as seasonal flu can be; and, unlike seasonal flu, it will be highly lethal. Concern over avian flu is also built on media hype. In 2005 and 2006, reporters and media pundits were able to elicit, from otherwise perfectly sane infectious disease experts, predictions that "an epidemic is inevitable; if not this year, then next." The late Dr. J. W. Lee, then the director general of the World Health Organization (WHO), was quoted by the Times on October 11, 2005: "The burning question is, will there be a human influenza pandemic? On behalf of WHO, I can tell you that there will be."

Yes, a deadly pandemic is probably inevitable, but whether it will occur during this decade or even the next is impossible to predict.[5]

Germs Responsible for "Noninfectious" Diseases

Among all the recently discovered aspects of human infection, one amazes me most of all: over the past two decades, we've learned that many of the diseases I'd been taught had nothing to do with infectious agents are, in fact, caused by "microbes." These diseases are neither rare nor trivial. They include devastating neurological entities, such as "mad cow" or variant Creutzfeldt-Jakob disease, caused by a curious class of infectious agents called prions; many, if not most, cases of liver cancer, caused by infection with hepatitis virus and by chronic exposure to aflatoxin, a chemical released by fungi growing on grain (ground nuts and the like) that has been poorly stored under tropical conditions; gastritis, stomach ulcers, and stomach cancer, caused not by "type A" personality or work-related stress but by a bacterium, Helicobacter pylori; and virtually all instances of cervical cancer, caused by infection with oncogenic (cancer-causing) strains of HPV.

Knowing that these diseases are infectious in origin opens new opportunities for their prevention (public health's Holy Grail). My two favorites (as exemplars of the breed) are H. pylori and HPV. When I trained in internal medicine, gastritis and ulcers were caused by "too much acid" and a "type A" personality. Aside from psychiatric counseling (not my provenance), patients were given tons of antacids; when they nonetheless arrived in the emergency ward at 3:00 a.m. with "black, tarry stools" (from bleeding, high in their bowels), we transfused pints of blood to make up for their loss, until such time as the surgeons could arrive to cut their vagus nerves (to reduce acid production) or whack out a large part of their stomach. Now, many such patients are cured with an antibiotic!

Scientists scoffed when Barry Marshall, an Australian physician, first proposed that H. pylori might be an important cause of gastritis and stomach ulcers. Only after he downed a flask full of the bacteria, duplicating the disease (and nearly killing himself in the process), did the medical community take notice. It is fortunate that he survived his experiment; it changed medical practice, and in the end he received the recognition (and compensation) he deserved, in the form of the 2005 Nobel Prize.

HPV makes for an equally compelling story, and its impact on the public's health may prove even greater. U.S. women well know the threat of cervical cancer. It is the reason they undergo regular, periodic Pap smears. The test is meant to detect early changes in cervical cells that herald the future development of invasive and deadly cancer. The test works well (for those who get it); early surgical intervention has drastically reduced the number of women dying each year from cervical cancer in the United States and other wealthy nations (poor people in the United States and people in poor countries remain at high risk of full-fledged cancer, disability, and death).

Within the past two decades, we've learned that virtually all cervical cancer in the world is the result of infection with a sexually transmitted virus: the human papilloma virus (HPV). HPV comes in many strains, some that cause cancer and some that don't. Most infections, regardless of strain, are readily cleared by the body without doing lasting damage. But when chronic infection occurs with an oncogenic strain, the stage is set for malignant alterations and subsequent cancer.[6]

If regular Pap smears and surgical intervention can prevent cervical cancer and death, what difference does the discovery of its infectious origins make? By detecting chronic infections with oncogenic strains, years before Pap smears become positive, the period between Pap smears can be safely extended, resulting in less-frequent tests. More important, new vaccines can now prevent infection and thereby prevent cancer in the first place. These vaccines are extremely effective; they can prevent infection by the two most common oncogenic strains of HPV, responsible between them for 75 percent of cancer and precancerous changes in U.S. women. It should be only a matter of time before improved vaccines can prevent infection from more strains of HPV, responsible for nearly 100 percent of all cervical cancer. Our granddaughters or, at the latest, their granddaughters will never need a Pap smear.

Populations currently too poor to receive regular Pap smears will benefit even more. Great clinical insights and epidemiology established the cause of this cancerous disease, great laboratory work produced its first vaccines, and great immunization programs could one day rid the world of a disease responsible for so much human suffering. But to be effective, immunization programs need to reach most girls and, ideally, boys as well, before they become sexually active (which is how they become infected). Why boys, when the purpose is to prevent cervical cancer? Because HPV, like HIV (and syphilis, herpes, and gonorrhea), is sexually transmitted. Girls might be the ones at risk of cervical cancer, but it's the boys who cause them to become infected.

In the United States, protests by parents, pastors, and politicians have stymied mandatory immunization in some locales. A common claim is that freedom from the fear of cervical cancer might increase promiscuity! Most children have absolutely no idea what a specific vaccine prevents, whether it is tetanus, diphtheria, measles, or chickenpox. It is absurd to think that one of many vaccines given to young girls would profoundly affect their subsequent sexual proclivities. The only thing these objections have done is raise the risk that some girls, not immunized when they should have been, might one day contract a deadly disease that could have been prevented.

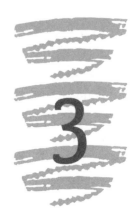

GENES

Sometimes "Destiny," Sometimes Not

So much has been written about the future benefits of the "genetic revolution" that it is left to me to play the Grinch. A little balance and reality testing are in order.

Genes are important, but not nearly as important as the media and NIH funding priorities would have us believe. They may be "destiny," but for the most part genes do not determine our state of health. If they did, how could life expectancy have doubled over the past century? We did not alter our genome dramatically during that short period of time.

The biggest thing we've learned from decoding the genome is that biological processes are infinitely more complicated than had been thought. Humans have far fewer genes than had been imagined; these somehow make more proteins and pieces of proteins than initially seemed possible. These proteins, genes, bits of genes, and even dark stretches once thought to be "genetic junk" signal one another in impossibly complex ways that modulate and regulate cellular functioning. Thus far, I am describing the complexity of a single cell, not a complex organism as intricate as humans. As Ludwig Wittgenstein once said about vision, "We find certain things about seeing puzzling because we do not find the whole business of seeing puzzling enough."[1] If seeing is a complicated function, imagine the complexity of the systems responsible for all of human functioning, health, and life!

Future research will reveal a great deal more about how cells and genes work, which is a good thing. Those doing that research are on an exciting ride. For the rest of us, the important point about genes for the moment is that most major diseases are influenced by the complex interactions between many genes (and other molecular and cellular elements) and our "environment." Many of the diseases in which genes probably play a role can be prevented now, without our knowing anything more about how genes function or awaiting the development of tools and techniques needed to change someone's genetic makeup.

Genes operate within the context we provide. If a Japanese man immigrates to the United States, his risk of stomach cancer plummets while his risk of heart disease skyrockets. He did not change his genes while flying across the Pacific. What he changed was the environment in which his genes now operate—principally, his diet. The high risk of stomach cancer in Japan is thought to be related to a diet rich in cured foods. The high risk of cardiovascular disease in the United States is related, at least in part, to a diet rich in salt and fats.

We stimulate our epidemiology students each year with this provocative thought: "In a country where everyone smokes, lung cancer would be considered a genetic disease." Most people my age know someone who smoked two packs of cigarettes a day and never developed lung cancer. We also know people who smoked "only" half a pack a day and got cancer. This suggests genetic variability in the risk of developing lung cancer from smoking. A "genetic" orientation to prevention would emphasize the need to find lung cancer–causing genes and innovative ways to block their effects. As best we know, this will take years of additional research. Alternatively, people could simply stop smoking!

I was dramatically reminded of these two different approaches to prevention while serving on a panel looking into "The Future of Medicine and Public Health." We had presented our thoughts at an evening session of the annual meeting of the American Public Health Association. People nodded politely and then left for dinner. A few months later, we repeated the exercise at the annual meeting of the American Medical Association. Just a few days earlier, the media had widely reported the discovery of a molecule in tobacco smoke that hooked up to the P53 gene, which might explain how smoking causes lung cancer. This report initially dominated the evening's discussion. While I found the report intellectually stimulating, I didn't believe it represented a major public health breakthrough. A member of the audience thought differently: "Now that we know what the receptor site looks like, the pharmaceutical industry can design a drug to block the offending molecule."

"Let me see if I understand what you are suggesting: we tell everyone to take a red pill every time they light up?"

"Exactly!"

"Even if that were possible, what do we do about smoking-induced heart disease, stroke, emphysema, chronic bronchitis, and bladder cancer? Have them also take yellow, blue, orange, green, and purple pills?"

The encounter taught us an important lesson: our panel abandoned its original notion that, to bridge the gap between "medicine" and "public health," all we needed to do was to train medical students to think like public health professionals. No public health professional would ever have thought the cure to an environmentally dependent disease was the formulation and ingestion of more pills; instead, the solution would reside in changing the environment.

Genetic screening plays an important role in identifying relatively uncommon but disastrous metabolic diseases, some of which we can mitigate. U.S. children are now routinely screened at birth for phenylketonuria. If positive, they are placed on a low-phenylalanine diet, which protects them from what otherwise would have been certain mental retardation.

Jews of European extraction (Ashkenazim) are at particularly high risk of a rare but deadly neurological disease, Tay-Sachs disease. Tay-Sachs disease occurs only if the fetus receives the defective gene, TSD, from both its parents. Voluntary screening can identify couples in whom each partner carries the gene and pinpoint their conceptions for further testing. By voluntarily identifying and aborting affected fetuses, Jewish couples in the United States have reduced the number of children born with Tay-Sachs disease by 90 percent. Among ultraorthodox communities in Israel, for whom procreation is important and abortion is prohibited, screening is done on older children. Rabbinical approval is withheld from those marriages that would unite two carriers of the mutant TSD gene.

Some of the most immediate and dramatic benefits of the genetic revolution have been new tools that identify individuals at dramatically increased risk of serious diseases we can do something about. Women carrying mutations in the BRCA1 and BRCA2 genes, for example, are at particularly high risk of developing breast cancer. But discovering that they carry the gene often leads to agonizing decisions—should they have frequent examinations but risk the chance that breast cancer won't be found early enough to cure, or should they undergo bilateral mastectomy at an early age (which does not entirely remove the risk of cancer)? The vast majority of women who develop breast cancer do not carry either of these BRCA mutations.

Sometimes knowing your risk of developing a disease can prove excruciatingly painful. It is now possible to identify nearly everyone who will one day develop Huntington disease, a devastating neurological condition whose onset is often not until midlife. If one parent has had the disease, the chance that an offspring carries the genetic defect and will be afflicted is 50:50. Because there is currently nothing we can do to prevent the disease, only 20 percent of those who know they are at potential risk of having the defect bother undergoing genetic testing; the other 80 percent have apparently concluded that they will discover their fate soon enough.

"Racial" variations in the risk of disease can sometimes reflect underlying genetic differences. Because sickle cell disease is due to a single mutated gene that arose in Africa, the disease is largely limited to those of African descent. But defining "race" can be tricky. Does it depend on skin pigmentation, one's friends or community, lifestyle, culinary preferences, language, or taste in music? In the last census, many Americans self-identified with more than one "race."

Knowing that some groups are at higher risk of developing a disease than others can help us identify the disease earlier in its course, thereby reducing the severity of its consequences. Higher risk does not necessarily mean, however, that the difference is genetic or even very large. For reasons we do not understand but suspect are at least partially genetic, African Americans are at four times greater risk of developing open-angle glaucoma than are Caucasians, and African Americans develop the disease at an earlier age. The American Academy of Ophthalmology and the National Eye Institute (of the National Institutes of Health) advocate earlier and more frequent glaucoma screening for African Americans. This is helpful, but we are a long way from knowing all the genetic markers for the disease and from having the ability to precisely pinpoint those needing added attention.

Some groups without shared genetic mutations are at increased risk of disease for totally different reasons. The poor are at increased risk of heart disease and stroke because of inadequate care of their hypertension and diabetes. "Men having sex with men" are at increased risk of HIV/AIDS (early in the epidemic in the United States, it was nearly unique to them) not because of their genetic makeup but because of their sexual proclivities.

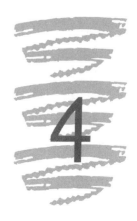

The Complex Nature of Causality

Disease and health are the outcome of complex, intersecting influences. Genes might vary the risk of lung cancer among smokers, but if you don't smoke, it is far less likely that you will get lung cancer. That's pretty straightforward. Other chains of causality are not.

We are experiencing global epidemics of asthma, diabetes, and heart disease. People have not changed their genes; what they've changed, broadly speaking, is their "environment": what they eat, what they drink, what they breathe, how they have sex, where they work—and with whom. Increased air pollution and more exposure to household dust and mites have raised the global risk of asthma. Jim Anthony, a professor of mental health at Johns Hopkins, has shown that asthma leads to "panic attacks." His colleague Bill Eaton has shown that panic attacks increase the risk of suicide. Finding proof might be difficult, but it seems reasonable to conclude that air pollution increases the number of suicides!

As for the "chaotic complexity of whole body biology," Matt Ridley points out in *Genome* that "stress" (as brought on, perhaps, by taking the college board exams) causes a whole cascade of physiological events, including increased levels of circulating cortisol, which influences the activity of the TFG gene on chromosome 10, suppressing the expression of interleukin 2 and thereby increasing the risk of infection.[1] Hence, taking an examination might indeed make you ill (something students have long claimed)!

Psychic Stressors

Some powerful determinants of health work through subtle psychological mechanisms. Michael Marmot, a respected English epidemiologist, provided one of the earliest and best illustrations of the "social gradient of disease." In his famous Whitehall Study, he followed the lives of London-based bureaucrats (who worked at Whitehall). He divided them into four social classes: the "born-to-lead" class (my terminology), scions of the upper classes who attended the "right" schools; the "professional and executive" class, who, being technocrats, were probably at least as well educated as the "born-to-lead" class (and perhaps more so); the clerical class; and "others." All were reasonably well paid by British standards, and all had the same access to the National Health Service.

What Marmot discovered should jolt anyone unfamiliar with his results: over the first ten years of follow-up, the "born-to-lead" class was the least likely to die, the professional and executive class had the next lowest death rate, and so forth. The differences were not trivial: the (well-educated) professional and executive class died at almost twice the rate of those "born to lead"; "others" died at more than three times the rate (Figure 10). In addition to differences in smoking, drinking, exercise, etc., there is something about one's class or standing in the social (pecking) order that dramatically affects health and survival. We don't yet know what it is; some have

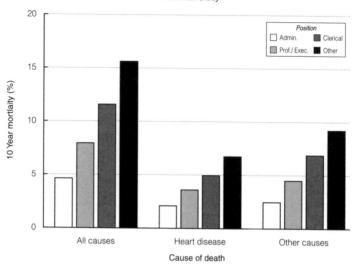

Age Adjusted Mortality Rates
Whitehall Study

Mortality rate among individuals working in the British bureaucracy, London. Over ten years of follow-up, those in the higher social classes died at lower rates than those "beneath" them. This was true for both cardiovascular and noncardiovascular causes of death. *Source*: Reprinted by permission from M. G. Marmot, "Social Differentials in Health between Populations," *Daedalus* 123 (1994): 202.

made a claim for self-efficacy (the ability to regulate one's own time and work), but we don't really know. Whatever the mechanism, it is unlikely to represent a new class of microbes or genes, but its influence seems to be no less determinate.

OUR "ENVIRONMENT"

It is widely accepted that our health (and a lot else about us) is determined by the interaction of our genes with our environment. But what is meant by *environment*? For a simple-minded person like me, it represents the constellation of factors that surround us (and our genes) and the medium by which they are transmitted (in the broadest terms, "infect" us). For example, the environment contains germs that are harmful to our health. They may be transmitted and infect us through the air we breathe, the food we eat, the water we drink, or by our turning the knobs on stateroom doors of luxury cruise ships (the way norovirus has ruined the holiday experiences of many a tourist).

Physical agents need not be germs. The great London smog of 1952 was responsible for an estimated twelve thousand deaths, simply because all that particulate matter in the air interfered with breathing. Dickens painted the classic picture of dark and "foggy" London without fully appreciating its effects on health. Because of strict regulations enacted after the deadly 1952 smog, Londoners can no longer warm their homes by burning coal in picturesque Edwardian fireplaces. The dramatic improvement in air quality prompted the British government to clean the walls of some of its most famous landmarks. I am still unnerved every time I visit London and rediscover that Big Ben, Parliament, and Westminster Cathedral were made of stone that is a golden brown—not black! Recently, sophisticated statistical modeling has shown that seemingly minor fluctuations in the amount of small particulate matter in the air of U.S. cities profoundly (if imperceptibly) affects our mortality.

Environments contain many toxic substances. As noted above (Chapter 2), aflatoxin, produced by a mold growing on ground nuts poorly stored under tropical conditions, "causes" liver cancer. Industrial toxicants of many types are accumulating in all the waters of the world. Some, a class called "endocrine disrupters," may be responsible for declining sperm counts in men in some regions and for increased risk of breast cancer and other reproductive abnormalities among women in others.

David Barker, an insightful English epidemiologist, was the first to suggest that things you are exposed to while in the womb might powerfully affect your future health. Enough evidence now supports this observation that "Barker's Hypothesis" has given way to a new field of investigation, "the fetal origins of adult disease." In essence, how you are nourished (or cared for) as a fetus and young infant alters the likelihood that you will develop diabetes or heart disease decades later. Presumably, these fetal factors "program" the future functioning of our genes and other cell-regulatory processes.

The environment also includes other "infectious" (if not microbial) agents that alter our health, including the marketing of pharmaceuticals and foods. Kelly Brownell, an innovative researcher at Yale, credits much of the obesity epidemic to our "toxic environment," an environment that engulfs us with inexpensive, enticing, high-calorie choices. The modest attack we've begun on childhood obesity strikes at the availability of high-calorie drinks and snacks in schools. In a famously dispiriting example, the Colorado School District signed a ten-year exclusivity contract with Coca-Cola. Only Coke products could be sold in their schools. In return, Coke agreed to give every elementary school $3,000, every middle school $15,000, and every high school $25,000. At first blush, it seemed that no harm had been done, a bonus for the schools for simply excluding Pepsi. Only later was it discovered that Coke's monetary grants depend on the school's achieving higher sales of beverages. When that did not occur, a deputy superintendent of the school system urged the principals to relax restraints on the purchase and use of Coke; he even encouraged them to allow students to drink cans of soda during class.

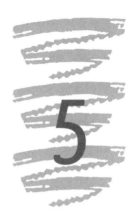

The Consequences
of Our Own Behavior

Many of our health problems are self-inflicted, things that we can do something about. One of "public health's" greatest modern triumphs was turning back the epidemic of cardiovascular disease that struck the United States after World War II. The epidemic peaked in the late 1950s, just before the great fuss over saturated fats and cholesterol in our diets. Army physicians were widely reported as being shocked by the levels of atherosclerosis they were seeing among teenage soldiers killed in Korea. Americans (on average) began to fret over their lipid levels and changed their diets. Over the ensuing thirty years, deaths from heart disease in the United States dropped by nearly half, long before potent lipid-lowering medications or bypass surgery was available (Figure 11).

Wealthy countries today have widely varying rates of death from heart disease. Hungary, Scotland, England, and Wales have some of the highest rates (Figure 12). This should be no surprise. As I explained to an audience at Trinity College, in Dublin, one had only to

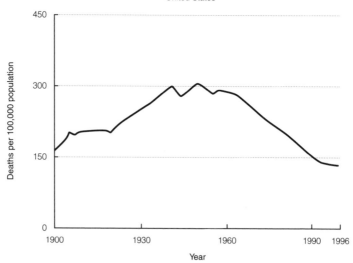

Death Rate from Heart Disease
United States

FIGURE 11. HEART DISEASE: A PUBLIC HEALTH TRIUMPH.
Death rate from heart disease in the United States, 1900–1996. U.S. death rates from heart disease, primarily coronary artery disease, reached a peak in the 1950s and have been falling ever since. This reflects the influence of better diets, more rigorous control of high blood pressure, and, recently, increasingly effective treatment options. Source: Adapted from Centers for Disease Control and Prevention, Morbidity and Mortality Weekly Report 48, no. 30 (August 6, 1999): 649, Figure 1.

reflect on what I'd been served for breakfast that morning: three fried eggs, sausage, ham, fried potatoes, fried tomatoes, and three pieces of toast soaked in butter. It was astonishing that I hadn't keeled over en route to the lecture hall!

THE USE OF TOBACCO

The U.S. epidemic of lung cancer has been even more dramatic than its epidemic of heart disease. U.S. women are understandably concerned about their risk of dying of breast cancer. Death rates from breast cancer were essentially unchanged from 1900 through 1990, though the picture has recently improved with more aggressive screening and earlier treatment, particularly with tamoxifen and other estrogen-blocking agents. At the same time, the risk for U.S. women of dying from lung cancer has skyrocketed! (See Figure 13.)

Virtually no U.S. women died of lung cancer in 1900; by 1940, large numbers of women had begun to die of lung cancer, but at only one-tenth the rate they died of breast cancer. By 1990, fifty years later, more U.S. women were dying from lung cancer than from breast cancer. Why? Because they'd "come a long way, baby." U.S. women first began to smoke in large numbers after World War I, and even more took up smoking after World War II. Their rates of lung cancer rose, as one would expect, after the twenty to thirty years it takes for lung cancer to develop.

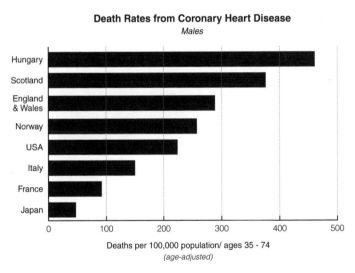

Death Rates from Coronary Heart Disease
Males

Deaths per 100,000 population/ ages 35 - 74
(age-adjusted)

FIGURE 12. WE ARE WHAT WE EAT.
Death rates for men from coronary artery disease in selected high-income countries. The death rates are highest in countries with diets rich in animal fats (Hungary, Scotland) and lowest where the diet is relatively low in animal fats (Japan).
Source: Adapted from D. Levy and W. B. Kannel, "Searching for Answers to Ethnic Disparities in Cardiovascular Risk," *Lancet* 356 (2000): 267.

The Consequences of Our Own Behavior   39

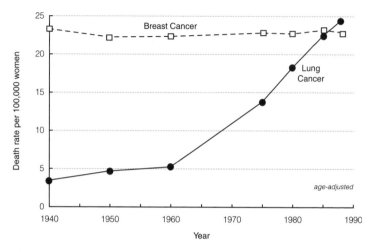

Female Cancer Death Rates
United States

FIGURE 13. WHAT'S WRONG WITH THIS PICTURE?
Deaths of women from breast and lung cancer in the United States, 1940–1990.
Between 1940 and 1990, an American woman's risk of dying from breast cancer
barely changed. In contrast, her risk of dying from lung cancer skyrocketed
because growing numbers of women began smoking after the two world wars. By
1990, more U.S. women were dying from lung cancer than from breast cancer.
Source: Adapted from D. Satcher, *Surgeon General's Report: Women and Smoking* (2001).

I've never understood why American women still passionately
organize "races for the cure" of breast cancer but seem indifferent
to a preventable disease that kills more of them. Of course, something along the same lines could be said of men (Figure 14).

Lung cancer is only one of the deadly consequences of smoking.
Add to it greatly increased rates of emphysema, chronic bronchitis,
cardiovascular disease (stroke and heart attacks), and a variety of
other conditions. Smoking is responsible for at least 400,000 excess
deaths in the United States every year. The numbers for Europe,
Japan, and the rest of the developed world dwarf our own. By 2050,
China, whose population has only recently taken up the addiction,
is expected to have 3 million excess deaths every year.

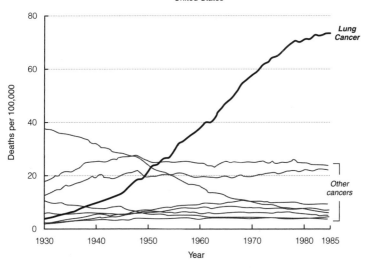

FIGURE 14. MEN ARE NO BETTER—IN FACT, THEY ARE WORSE.
Cancer death rates of men in the United States, 1930–1985. Death rates from lung
cancer among American men have climbed steadily, while their risk of death from
most other forms of cancer has remained fairly flat or declined, reflecting their
long history of smoking. Source: Adapted from *Cancer Facts and Figures* (American Cancer
Society, 2008).

The United States has taken a global lead in reducing the use of
tobacco. Over the past two decades, smoking rates in the United
States have dropped from roughly half of all adults to barely one-
fourth. Some health benefits, such as a fall in asthma attacks among
children residing in the home of a smoker, have been almost immediate; others, such as diminishing rates of lung cancer and emphysema among smokers, will be slower to arrive as we experience the
chronic, long-term consequences of years of past smoking. But
these benefits will show up.

Four hundred years ago, King James complained that smoking
was "a custome loathsome to the eye, hateful to the nose, harmful
to the braine, (and) dangerous to the lungs." In 1938 Raymond Pearl,

professor of biostatistics at the Johns Hopkins School of Public Health, published dramatic data demonstrating that smokers died at a much younger age than nonsmokers. By 1954, Sir Richard Doll had confirmed the unique risk of lung cancer among smokers. On July 13, 1957, Leroy Bernie, the U.S. surgeon general (and an alumnus of the Hopkins School of Public Health), was quoted on the front page of the New York Times: "It is clear that there is an increasing and consistent body of evidence that excessive cigarette smoking is one of the causative factors in lung cancer." Why, then, did smoking in the United States only recently, if dramatically, decline? The eventual decline in tobacco use in the United States owes much to long-term advocacy on the part of antitobacco activists and to revelations, during health-related liability suits, of the cynical manipulations and bare-faced hypocrisy of the tobacco industry. Most important, smoking became socially unacceptable among large parts of society.

Thirty years ago, most Americans had ashtrays scattered about their homes, if not for themselves, then for guests. No longer. If you wanted to smoke at a winter dinner party at my home fifteen years ago, you went out in the cold. What empowered so many of us to become so rude? I suspect it was recognition of the dangers of "side-stream smoke." A nonsmoker who lives in the same home as a smoker is far more likely to develop tobacco-related illnesses than are nonsmokers who live in homes where nobody smokes. No longer did smoking harm only the smoker; your smoking not only smelled up my living room but also increased my chance of death (and my child's risk of asthma).

The remaining challenge for the United States is to reduce the use of tobacco among the 25 percent of adults who still smoke and, most important, to reduce the risk that young people will start to smoke. Most adult smokers began smoking as teenagers; once you are a smoker, stopping is hard to do.[1]

Michael Bloomberg, the mayor of New York City, and his activist commissioner of health, Tom Frieden, used this powerful argument in their effective campaign against smoking. Their three-pronged attack: dramatically raise the cost of cigarettes by imposing an additional three dollar tax per pack, making them less affordable to teenagers; use the funds raised by that tax for aggressive counteradvertising—educating the public about the harms of smoking (and, at least as important, about why taxes were raised and other reforms introduced); and outlaw smoking in bars and restaurants. The last proved the most contentious: owners of bars and restau-

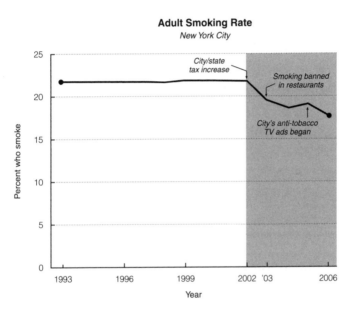

Adult Smoking Rate
New York City

FIGURE 15. GOVERNMENT-DIRECTED SMOKING CESSATION EFFORTS CAN WORK.
Adult smoking rates, New York City. A decline in the number of adults who smoke followed each New York City intervention: a dramatic increase in the tax (and therefore the cost) of cigarettes; banning smoking in bars and restaurants; and counteradvertising that dramatically illustrated the health consequences of smoking. Source: Data from the Centers for Disease Control and Prevention, *Morbidity and Mortality Weekly Report* 56, no. 24 (June 22, 2007): 604–8.

TABLE 1. SMOKING RATES, BY AGE GROUP, IN NEW YORK CITY,
2002 AND 2006

Age Group	Percentage Who Smoke	
	2002	2006
18–24	23.8	15.5
25–44	24.3	20.2
45–64	23.4	19.2
65+	10.0	9.9
Overall	21.6	17.5
	= 19% reduction overall	

Source: Data from Morbidity and Mortality Weekly Report 56, no. 24 (June 22, 2007): 604–8.

Note: After four years of New York City tobacco control initiatives, the percentage of adults who smoked dropped for every age group except among the small number of highly addicted survivors, 65 years or older. The greatest reduction in smoking prevalence occurred among the youngest age group—those who were the newest smokers or were dissuaded from smoking in the first place.

rants claimed that the ban infringed on the rights of drinkers and diners and would cost them business. The mayor's counterargument: he had no choice; this was all about occupational safety and health. People who worked in bars and restaurants had a right to a healthy work environment; smoking was inimical to workers' health.

The argument worked, and so did the program. Within two years, tobacco use in New York City declined by 15 percent (Figure 15). Even more encouraging were changes in the age-specific smoking rates (Table 1). The greatest reduction in smoking occurred among those 18 to 24 years of age, in whom the rate of smoking fell from 24 to 15 percent (a relative decline of 35 percent). Among those 20 through 65 years old, the rate of smoking fell from 24 to 19 percent. Among those over the age of 65, smoking rates didn't budge: 10 percent smoked before the program began and 10 percent smoked afterward. Ten percent smoked beforehand? Why not 24 percent, as in younger adults? Because these long-term smokers had died at more than twice the rate of nonsmokers. Those still alive were too badly hooked to quit. As a bonus, patronage of bars and restaurants rose! This was a uniquely instructional outcome. New York City's program is now being copied throughout Europe (even Ireland's famously smoky pubs are now smoke-free). "Big Tobacco" is banking on making up for its losses in Europe and the United States by boosting tobacco sales in the developing world. Mike Bloomberg (as philanthropist—not mayor) has already committed nearly $400 million to counter Big Tobacco's assault on the developing world. Last year Bill Gates joined him.[2]

OBESITY

The other great epidemic, obesity, is still in its infancy and will likely prove a lot harder to combat. Can food create an epidemic? The Centers for Disease Control and Prevention (CDC) has been "tracking" the rates of overweight and obesity in the United States. Between 1991 and 1998, the number of states in which 15 percent or more of the adult population was obese grew like wildfire (Figure 16). By 2008, more than one-quarter of all U.S. adults, and 40 percent of all African American women, were obese; another third were clinically overweight. The epidemic now circles the globe, engulfing rich and poor nations alike. The number of Australian schoolchildren who are overweight doubled, from 12 to 24 percent, in just three years. The number of overweight English pre–school age children rose from 15 to 24 percent in a decade. Dacca, the capital of Bangladesh, where my family and I lived among famously skinny Bengalis from 1970 through 1972, now sports McDonald's, Pizza Hut, and other fast food outlets for the growing middle class— whose children are growing, indeed. On any weekend, increasingly plump adolescents can be seen rolling out of these restaurants' doors, incongruously mixing with the wizened rickshaw drivers and beggars in the streets.[3]

How did this happen? Very simply: we eat a great deal more today than we ever did before. Food in the United States has become

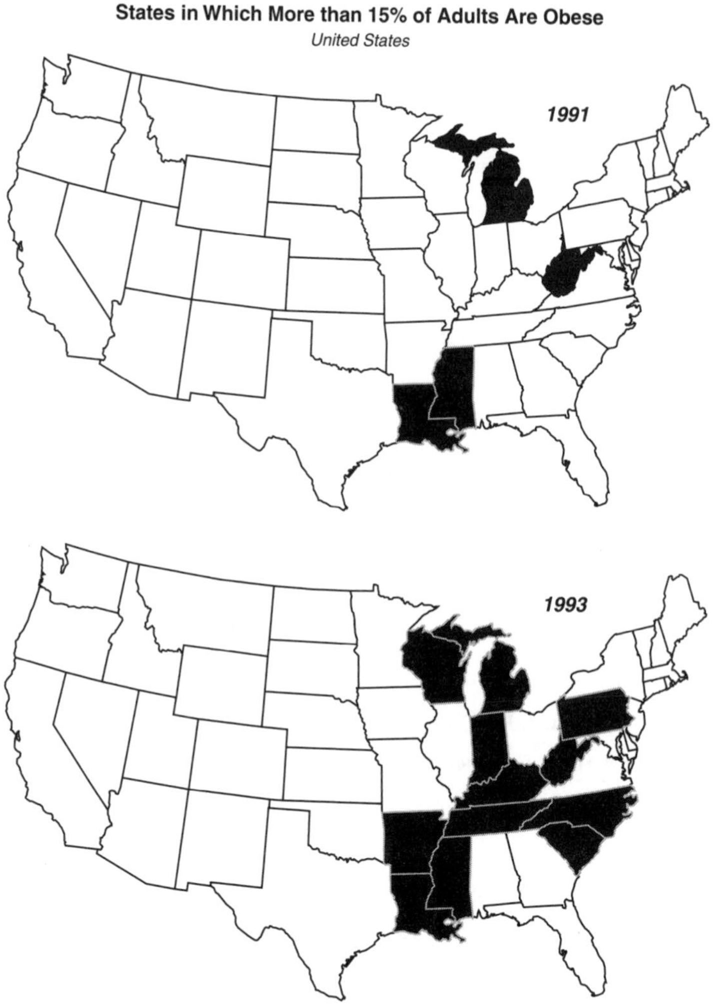

States in Which More than 15% of Adults Are Obese
United States

1991

1993

FIGURE 16. OBESITY AS AN "EPIDEMIC."
U.S. states in which more than 15 percent of adults are obese (a BMI of 30 or greater). Source: Reprinted by permission from Centers for Disease Control and Preven-

cheap; by some estimates, 8 percent of disposable income is spent on food in the United States versus 24 percent in Europe. Portion sizes have gotten larger. And, of course, we began to "supersize." The origins of supersizing are well told in Eric Schlosser's Fast Food

States in Which More than 15% of Adults Are Obese
United States

1995

1998

tion, Behavioral Risk Factor Surveillance System: U.S. Obesity Trends, 1915–2006 (www.cdc
.gov/nccdphp/dnpa/obesity/trend/maps/index.htm).

Nation. Marketing gurus discovered that it was a lot easier to sell
one large portion than to convince people to buy two regular-sized
portions. The economics were compelling. The cost of most fast
foods is not in the calories it contains but in its preparation, packag-

ing, and delivery. A large Coke costs the retailer an extra 3 cents for syrup but is sold for 20 cents more than the smaller size. The net profit: an additional 17 cents per purchase.

Between 1990 and 2000, we Americans increased our food consumption by 8 percent, an astounding 140 extra pounds of food per person per year! It's surprising that we are not even bigger than we already are! By some calculations, nearly 80 percent of our increased caloric intake since 1977 has come from sweetened beverages ("fruit" juices and soda).

It's not only how much we eat but also what we eat. Some foods are far more "calorie-dense": fat, for example, contains many more calories per gram (or pound) than does protein. Pima Indians have a high rate of diabetes, which is closely linked to weight, and are therefore of particular interest to nutritionists. Pima Indians living on the Mexican side of the border consume a relatively traditional diet, in which fat comprises 23 percent of what they eat. On average, they have a relatively svelte body mass index of 25 (borderline "overweight"). The diet consumed by Pima Indians just across the border, in Arizona, contains 41 percent fat; their average BMI is 37 (a BMI of 30 is "obese").

Simply deciding to "eat right" won't help much unless you have appropriate choices and information about the composition and quality of your food. Those who choose Chicken McNuggets rarely recognize that a serving contains twice the fat, per ounce, of a McDonald's hamburger. Are you eating at the tasty and (relatively) inexpensive Cheesecake Factory, and for health reasons you've decided to indulge in a slice of carrot cake instead of chocolate cheesecake? One slice of their carrot cake contains 1,600 calories, nearly a full day's caloric requirement.

The growth in overweight and obesity (pun intended) has already spurred the "resizing" of American and French women's wear—you might still wear the same "size" 6, but it is now a lot larger. My wife,

Jill, is rapidly approaching size "0" without ever having changed her weight.

Weight is not just an issue for fashionable women's wear: obesity is blamed for the rapidly spreading epidemic of diabetes among children and adults alike, with all the health consequences that go along with the disease: blindness, kidney failure, heart disease, neurological complications, and amputations. When I trained in medicine, non-insulin-dependent diabetes (NIDDM) was also labeled "adult onset." No longer. It is now a regular occurrence among adolescents (and their even younger siblings). Their genes haven't changed.

No one has yet discovered an effective way to stop the obesity epidemic—at least, not a way consistent with our freedoms and standard of living. Though you might crowd my airline seat and raise the average cost of health care in the United States, your obesity, unlike side-stream tobacco smoke, won't kill me. Most of us have been taught since childhood to be respectful of those who are fat. And, as the powerful agricultural industry is quick to point out, "We're not tobacco; you can't demonize food."

A note of advice to the concerned reader: if you don't want to gain weight, eat less! No one (since last lectured by one's mother) insists that you "finish everything on your plate." Our plates have gotten way too large for a normal, healthy diet. Exercise is good for a lot of reasons, but losing weight is not one of them. Warding off the effects of that single slice of carrot cake would require running eighteen miles—and not ending up being so hungry that you return for another slice.[4]

Changing behaviors is hard, particularly at the individual level. Most people don't operate in isolation. We reflect the values, preferences, and norms of the people we most admire and with whom we identify and associate (Figure 17). These social networks are powerful determinants of behavior: family and close friends; members of

**FIGURE 17. PEOPLE DON'T
ENTIRELY HAVE FREE WILL.**
Our choices and behavior are
influenced by the choices and
behavior of others, particularly
those within our social networks
(whether members of our family,
colleagues in our workplace, or
the wider community at large).

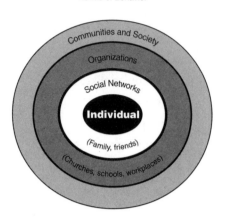

Social Determinants
Norms of Behavior

our church, other students at school, and colleagues in our work-place; others in our community; and society at large. We are a product of their expectations and their behavior; it is what defines us as being part of our "clan." Fewer than 10 percent of all adult immigrants to the United States are obese on arrival; by the time they have lived here fifteen years, they've caught up with the rest of us (Figure 18). A recent study showed that those who become obese are far more likely to know people who are obese—the media joked that obesity seems to be infectious (in a sociological sense, it is).

To change most people's behavior, we need to change the norms of their clan. That's easy to say! A group of classes were "educated" about the dangers of smoking from the third through the tenth grades. After fifteen years of education and follow-up, one-quarter smoked, exactly the same rate as among the controls. Adults told that they were at genetically high risk of developing smoking-related cancers kept smoking at the same rate as those who were not at increased risk. As reported in 2001 by Research!America, according to Louis Sherwood, then a leading laboratory scientist at Merck & Co., a pharmaceutical company, "A lot of what we are talking about in prevention is behavioral change. I can assure you that it is a lot easier to do molecular biology." Or, as Steve Jones put it in the Milbank Fund, "Genetics has little relevance to the treatment of NIDDM [type 2, non-insulin-dependent diabetes]; banning cheese-burgers would do far more good."[5]

The war on tobacco was successful to the degree that it changed societal norms. We hadn't suddenly discovered that smoking was bad for us. When my teenage friends and I experimented with smoking fifty years ago, we asked one another for "a coffin nail." It was not as if we didn't know that smoking was unhealthy! My

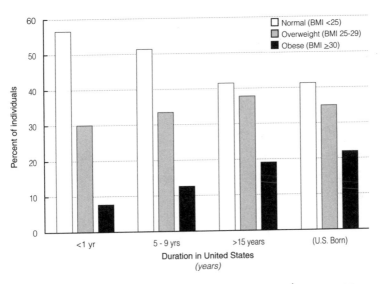

Change in Weight of U.S. Immigrants

FIGURE 18. PEOPLE NOT OBESE OFTEN BECOME OBESE (LIKE THOSE AROUND THEM).

Change in weight among U.S. immigrants. Upon arrival in the United States, immigrants are less likely to be obese than are native-born Americans. After fifteen years of residence, however, their risk of obesity more than doubles, catching up to those who were native born. Source: Adapted from M. S. Gael, E. P. McCarthy, R. S. Phillips, et al., "Obesity among U.S. Immigrant Subgroups by Duration of Residence," *Journal of the American Medical Association* 292 (2004): 2865.

favorite internist routinely counseled his patients to eat right and avoid cigarettes; he himself was an obese smoker.[6]

TREATMENT IS TOUGH; PREVENTION IS TOUGHER

Some prevention strategies are relatively easy to implement and are highly effective: sanitation and clean water, vaccination, cars with "crumple zones." What makes them effective is that the individual is a relatively passive recipient of the strategy's benefits. One measles immunization at the appropriate age, and it is unlikely you'll ever get measles. If you live in a major U.S. city, it is practically impossible to catch a water-borne infection. Your car's "crumple zones" absorb the energy of a collision, reducing the risk of serious roadway injury.

But reducing smoking, obesity, and HIV requires changing personal preferences and behaviors, giving up today's pleasures (sex, tobacco, chocolate, a 1982 Bordeaux) for some theoretical health benefit long in the future. Because the health benefit is a "non-event" (you didn't have your first heart attack at age forty-eight or get smallpox), it isn't even noticed.

As we've seen with tobacco, changes in societal norms can change individual preferences and behavior. The most efficient and effective tools for changing societal behavior are the five "shuns": education, regulation, taxation, legislation, and litigation. Education is important, but mostly for informing people why the four other powerful arbiters of behavior are being deployed. Knowing that second-hand smoke kills eventually moved politically effective leaders to ban smoking from public places, impose draconian taxes on tobacco products, regulate the addicting constituents of cigarettes, and take the tobacco companies to court. Public health is a public good; effective change almost always requires political action and support.

But many health decisions, particularly those that need to be made individually, are less susceptible to societal pressures or political intervention. Education helps; so does repetition and not-so-subtle reinforcement. Tom Frieden, as New York City's activist health commissioner (he's now director of the CDC), waged a successful battle to force restaurant chains to display the caloric content of every item as prominently as they display its price. If the customer is reminded that a piece of delicious, inexpensive carrot cake contains a full day's caloric needs, he or she might be inclined to split it with a friend. The "toxic environment" that Kelly Brownell credits with promoting the overeating responsible for obesity can be mitigated by a myriad of small gestures—for example, omitting high-calorie snacks (potato chips, M&Ms, and sweetened drinks) from conference tables removes much of the inducement to snack during meetings.

We sometimes advise people to do things they simply cannot do. "Eat a balanced diet" (whatever that means) is probably good advice, particularly when backed up with practical suggestions. But poor, inner-city populations often lack access to "healthy" foods: local markets don't carry fresh vegetables and fish, and when they do, they are much more expensive than fast foods. Fried foods may be not only your cultural norm but also all that's available and all you can afford.

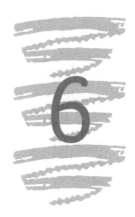

Choosing the Healthier Lifestyle

To choose healthier behaviors, we need to know what makes and keeps us healthy. Unfortunately, much of what we are told simply isn't true. Researchers overinterpret their data; medical journals, in a competition to be quoted, overstate the relevance of the results; and anchors on the evening news seek out the most sensational stories. Data are hyped to the third power! What we don't learn from the evening news, we learn from the drug company ads that sustain them. These are meant to sell drugs to people who largely don't need them.

What I can't explain is why Americans seem (uniquely) mesmerized by "medical" news or why, like lemmings, we are so quick to embrace purportedly healthy interventions. (Remember the proliferation of "low-carb" products that briefly swamped our supermarket shelves?)

First, why is the latest medical "news" so regularly unreliable? For at least four reasons: The first is the need to attract readers and primetime viewers. "Breakthroughs" and "miracles" sell. Editors routinely advise would-be letter and opinion writers to make their communications counterintuitive, novel, and, above all, controversial. Reporters have heard the same advice. The more off-beat and outlandish the claim, the larger the headline (and more likely the byline).

The second factor stems from competition among medical journals to be referenced in the lay media. Too many medical editors seek out manuscripts they believe will make headlines and employ staff whose purpose is to ensure that they do. When I made this observation to Larry Altman, the respected former senior medical writer of the New York Times, he replied, "Really Al, why do you think they are called 'medical journals'? They are run by 'journalists.'"

What's scary is that the public are not the only ones who get their medical education from the lay press. Medical experts are more likely to take notice of articles in their own field that have been cited in the New York Times! For example, articles published in the New England Journal of Medicine are nearly twice as likely to be referenced by other scientists once they've been mentioned in the New York Times. This appears to have little to do with either the value of the article or its subject matter: research reports were as likely to be overlooked by fellow scientists when the Times chose to ignore the research as when the Times couldn't possibly take notice because it was on strike.

The third factor is the proclivity of some medical researchers to claim more than their study proves. Too often, huge importance is given to tiny but tantalizing bits of new data. Not all medical researchers do this, but enough do. Being quoted on National Public Radio (NPR) rarely hurts future funding or academic advancement. It is also becoming more common (NIH funding these days is, unfortunately, a "zero-sum" game). For the most part, investigators carefully hedge extrapolated claims in their scientific publications by acknowledging the preliminary nature of their finding and the need to confirm its clinical relevance. But "preliminary" and "inconclusive" are not what the public wants to hear—and so they don't.

Sometimes "results" pile up in bizarre and confusing ways. One series of closely timed headlines can be summarized as follows: exercise reduces the risk of a subsequent heart attack; the risk of sudden death is increased sixteen-fold during vigorous exercise; this increased risk of death during exercise declines the more you exercise. If those conclusions don't confuse your plans for healthier living, add these: the risk of sudden death increases tenfold after a large meal; the size of that risk is about the same order of magnitude as the risk of sudden death associated with having sex; the increase in the risk of death associated with a large meal disappears two hours after the meal (I don't know how long after having sex). I'm not certain any of this is true, but I am certain the average lay reader would find it easy to dismiss. As Voltaire once said, "Common sense is not so common."

The last cause for confusion is the nature of the research being reported. The discovery of some new metabolic pathway or cellular receptor site might be the ticket to a Nobel Prize, but rarely does it carry sufficient drama to make the front page. "Epidemiological" research, on the other hand, can be (and often is) hyped to the hills. Being an epidemiologist, I find this particularly galling.

Two types of epidemiological studies dominate clinical insights and the evening news. One, the randomized clinical trial, is often definitive. Individuals are randomly assigned to one of two interventions, and the outcomes are compared. Done correctly, and with a modicum of luck, one intervention proves dramatically superior to the other. Because the intervention should be the only factor that differed between the two groups, one can reasonably conclude that the intervention was responsible for the difference in outcomes.

The other type of epidemiological study is entirely observational. The researcher observes how people lead their lives and then notes what happens to them. The investigator has no control over the factors of interest or the patient's outcome. All he or she can do is calculate the rate at which an outcome of interest occurs in people who differ in many ways. Did people who lived longer eat more salad, run three miles a day, prefer apples to pears, have more (or less) sex, or beat their dog?

Observational studies often identify factors that appear to be associated with better health. But "association" is not "causality." These clues need far more proof before entering the medical canon. Why? Because people differ, in more ways than the preference for apples or pears. Those who live longer might well prefer apples but might also run two miles a day, never have sex, eat Cheerios for breakfast, sleep eight hours a night, use a specific multivitamin supplement, smoke a pipe, leave their window ajar in the evening, and keep cats. Or they might not.

When the news claims that a specific factor observed to be "associated" with a clinical outcome was the "cause" of the disease, the epidemiologist will commonly have claimed to have "adjusted for all other differences." That is silly. Statistical adjustments are often complex, "black-box" mathematical affairs entailing numerous, inadequately tested assumptions, most of which the average epidemiologist isn't even aware of. The biggest assumption is that the study collected data on the most important characteristics in the first place! Because one rarely knows what those are at the outset, it's hard to be certain they were collected—assuming it is even possible to collect them. Complex mental processes and fleeting molecular interactions defy collection.

Extrapolations of simple, observed associations are the commonest reason we are warned one day that coffee "causes" pancreatic cancer or heart disease and a few weeks later that it doesn't. One memorable headline announced: "Coffee might help to prevent gallstones, but hold decaf."

Sometimes the studies were designed differently. Sometimes they ask different questions of different data. Sometimes the populations under study are different in ways that even the investigators never grasp.

The conflicting "results," conclusions, and recommendations emanating from observational studies have not gone unnoticed. One opinion piece in the New York Times lampooned: "It's Good. No, It's Bad. No, It's Good. Really. I Think."[1]

John Terry followed suit in the Baltimore Sun: " 'OK,' said the chairman, Al [I'm certain he was not referring to me—but that, too, is an untested hypothesis]. 'Let's summarize what we know. We know that you need vitamins, but high dosages may not be any better for you than low doses. Maybe worse, in fact. Or maybe not.' 'I move that we declare low doses of vitamins A through G, medium doses of vitamins H through R, and high doses of vitamins S through Z good for you,' said Margaret. 'Or bad for you. Whichever.'"[2]

Many observational studies have suggested that people who eat salad, particularly salads rich in beta-carotene, are less likely to develop cancer. This association was so ubiquitous in observational studies that it had practically become an article of faith that beta-carotene prevented most major forms of cancer. Fortunately, this conclusion was subjected to randomized trials. In each instance, participants assigned to consume pills stuffed with extra beta-carotene experienced more lung cancer than those consuming the placebo. Beta-carotene supplements increased the risk of lung cancer among smokers and did nothing to reduce it among nonsmokers.

Randomized trials have overturned other "truths" underlying advice for "healthy living"—"truths" based primarily on evidence from nonrandomized observational studies. Not too long ago, we were told that dietary "roughage" (fiber) was important for good health. Perhaps it is. But one specific claim, that it prevented colon cancer, proved, in a carefully conducted randomized trial, not to be true.

For years I took an inexpensive multivitamin pill each morning, primarily to get extra folic acid. Why? Because knowledgeable colleagues insisted that folic acid reduced the risk of heart attack—some had even criticized federal authorities for not advocating this practice. What was the basis for this strongly held belief? Primarily two observations: children born with a metabolic defect that results in high levels of homocysteine develop atherosclerosis at an early age, and folic acid depresses homocysteine levels. Ergo, men (because men are at greater risk of early heart attack than are women) should take extra folic acid (only those with elevated homocysteine levels might benefit, but these levels were hard to measure, and no one really knows what constitutes an "elevated" level). I stopped taking my daily vitamin pill when randomized trials of folic acid (with and without other B vitamins) failed to demonstrate any reduction in the risk of heart attack. Another worthless "healthy habit."

Folic acid also provides a contrasting story—with a decidedly happier outcome. A set of observational studies suggested that low levels of folic acid, early in pregnancy, increased the risk of neurologically devastating (and often fatal) congenital neural tube defects, such as spina bifida. Population-based trials proved that increasing folic acid intake before conception reduces this risk. The United States now mandates fortification of cereal grain meant for human consumption with folic acid to ensure that women have healthier levels of folic acid from the time of conception.

Because one can't do a randomized trial on everything of interest, "evidence" obtained from observational studies is sometimes stretched pretty far. A lot farther (and thinner) than it deserves.

A respected epidemiologist and nutritionist has been deeply involved with several unique, long-running observational studies. He is also a strong advocate for healthy living—advice that is largely based on the "associations" these studies have uncovered. But even I was startled to read in the New York Times that a new, nonabsorbable (therefore calorie-free) fat substitute to be used in preparing potato chips and other snacks would result in "2000 to 9,800 cases of prostate cancer, 32,000 additional cases of coronary heart disease, 1,400 to 7,400 excess cases of lung cancer, and 80 to 390 more cases of macular degeneration" every year. How did he know this? First, by estimating the number of excess cases of these diseases that might be "associated," in observational studies, with low intake of some fat-soluble nutrients (beta-carotene, vitamin A, etc.). He then assumed that the nonabsorbable fat substitute would further reduce the intake of these fat-soluble nutrients and by what amount. From this third-order assumption, he calculated the precise amount of unnecessary disease and death that would ensue. He organized a press conference on the subject and estimated, for the Times, the huge risk Americans would needlessly suffer. In fact, evidence that these fat-soluble substances protect us from these diseases is less than overwhelming; as in the case of beta-carotene and lung cancer, it might not even be true! Being an advocate for health, he forgot for the moment how imprecise and inconclusive his observations and assumptions were.

Sometimes everyone—the investigator, the medical journal, and the lay press—misinterprets the data. Not to gain publicity but simply because he or she wasn't thinking clearly. Two examples will suffice.

As an aging academic spending a good deal more than I should taking daily tablets of chondroitin sulfate to reduce the pain in my arthritic knees, I paid more than usual attention to an article on the subject that appeared in the Times. According to my favorite "newspaper of record," a randomized trial just published in the New England Journal of Medicine had conclusively shown that chondroitin sulfate provided little if any benefit. Curious, I read the original New England Journal article carefully. Sure enough, the authors concluded that chondroitin "did not reduce pain effectively in the overall group of patients with osteoarthritis of the knee." But, when the authors looked at the impact on different groups of patients in the study, they had to conclude that "exploratory analyses suggest ... [chondroitin sulfate] ... may be effective in the subgroup of patients with moderate to severe knee pain." Aha! You obtain pain relief only if you feel pain (or, at a minimum, moderate pain). I still take the pills, and they still seem to work.

Another recent trial concluded that supplemental calcium and vitamin D given to healthy postmenopausal women resulted in a small improvement in bone density but "did not significantly reduce hip fractures" (preventing hip fractures is an important reason for wanting dense bones). Near the end of the published report, I discovered an important caveat: among study participants who took the supplements at least 80 percent of the time, the risk of hip fracture fell by 30 percent. You have to take your supplement to benefit from it! Why wasn't that the story?

Sometimes well-conducted studies yield results requiring a sophisticated balancing of benefit and harm. Drugs that are lifesaving in one dose are toxic in another. But a new health discovery or recommendation, particularly one that is grist for the media mill, can't be subtle or nuanced. Raw emotions then decide.

The heavily funded and much-anticipated Women's Health Initiative conducted a large, randomized trial of the benefits and harms of hormone replacement therapy (HRT) for menopausal and postmenopausal women. The day it reported that women randomly assigned to take HRT had an "increased" number of heart attacks, the study was terminated (earlier than planned) and the stock price of the HRT pharmaceutical maker plummeted. Early termination was

TABLE 2. THE EFFECTS OF HORMONE REPLACEMENT THERAPY

Event	Number*
Detrimental effect	
Coronary event	+7
Stroke	+8
Embolus	+8
Breast cancer	+8
Beneficial effect	
Colorectal cancer	–6
Hip fracture	–5

Source: Data from Writing Group for the Women's Health Initiative Investigators, "Risks and Benefits of Estrogen Plus Progestin in Healthy Menopausal Women: Principal Results from the Women's Health Initiative Randomized Controlled Trial," *Journal of the American Medical Association* 288, no. 3 (2002): 321–33.
* "Excess" number of cases that occur each year among 10,000 women taking HRT.

probably appropriate. But the therapeutic implications of the data were more nuanced. For every ten thousand women taking HRT for one year, the investigators estimated there would be an additional seven coronary events (a rate of less than one-tenth of 1 percent) and eight strokes, pulmonary emboli, and cases of invasive breast cancer. But these same HRT users would benefit from six fewer instances of colorectal cancer and five fewer hip fractures. There was no difference in the overall risk of death between those taking HRT and those taking the placebo (Table 2).

How will this all end? The present trajectory suggests, not well. Tara Parker-Pope, of the *New York Times*, scathingly reviewed *The Fertility Diet*, a recent book by "Harvard researchers." Much of the advice was based on data from the Nurses Study, a long-running observational investigation following the habits and health of nurses who periodically report what they do and what they eat. Parker-Pope quotes one author as saying that it is "highly likely" that the diet recommendations will help some women become pregnant. On the other hand, he admitted that the Nurses Study "found associations between fertility and certain eating behaviors, but it didn't test whether adopting new eating habits would make a difference." Bravo! Round 1 goes to Parker-Pope's caution. So did round 2. When she explored the reasons for writing the book and the shallowness of the evidence on which it was based, the lead author explained, "It had been a challenge to balance the limitations of scientific research with the commercial demands of book publishing; even the simple title of the book, he added, belies the complexity of the findings."[3]

Need anyone wonder why the public is confused? The real mystery is why the public still cares!

Our other major source of medical information, the pharmaceutical industry, has an even greater proprietary interest: selling drugs. I can't help but notice that at least half the ads interspersed with the evening news are directed at me (or my wife). Viagra was an instant hit with baby boomers but only after the condition it treated, "erectile dysfunction," was invented as a way to medicalize what had previously been considered simply one more manifestation of aging (earlier in some, later in others, like most aging-related phenomena).

Who knew there was a medical condition called RLS (restless leg syndrome)? No one, until a pharmaceutical company discovered a "treatment" that allegedly relieves it. Or, as the makers of Zoloft enquire in a serene and moving ad, "Is she just shy, or is it Social Anxiety Disorder? Zoloft—Indicated for Social Anxiety Disorder." Were you a wallflower in high school or mentally ill?

Some pharmaceutical advertising is superficially more informative than others. Those that claim a specific medical benefit must also disclose all the potential complications, hazards, and side effects. Those that make no specific claims for their drug, need not. I suspect that explains why I can't forget the importance of asking my doctor whether "the purple pill" is right for me, while not having the slightest idea what it is for!

The informed consumer can, depending on what he or she has read and decided to believe, pursue a "Mediterranean diet," with its healthy grains and olive oil, or abhor it, as would any righteous Atkins dieter, knowing that "carbs" are the "true" source of global obesity. Those concerned that red meat (and its fats) promote atherosclerosis, heart disease, and stroke can switch to fish for its purportedly healthy omega-3 oils, but they best not be too concerned that environmental wastes have laden popular fish with mercury, PCBs, and other toxic chemicals.

When asked for guidance, most nutritionists and dietitians fall back on the old bromide, "Eat a balanced and varied diet; nothing in excess" (without telling you exactly what that means, how one puts it into practice, or what evidence underlies the recommendation). On a recent Lufthansa flight, my business class menu included an option called Flight Line "for our guests who value a light and balanced nutrition." My choices included grilled beef tenderloin ("in Merlot demiglace") as an entrée and cheesecake for dessert.

Where does this leave the concerned, conscientious, and would-be informed health consumer? Confused! But there are ways to stay on top of whatever is worth staying on top of.

First, disregard broadcasters' breathlessly communicated evening news. The anchor rarely provides more than a ten- or twenty-second sound bite. I often wonder whether the writers spend even that much time researching the issue. Have you noticed that all three major channels inevitably cover the same story and that you almost never hear about it again? It's as if broadcasters all work from the same playbook—which in a sense they do, because they were trained to find headline-grabbing items in the same ways. Ditto drug company ads and "infomercials." Overwhelmingly, these are designed for only one purpose: to get us to take drugs we probably don't need, often for conditions that don't exist!

Second, did the recommendation make it into a major newspaper, and, if so, how much space was it allotted, how many experts unrelated to the investigators were quoted, and how uniform were their "expert" opinions? None of this is proof that the claims are real, but the answers will help to winnow down the field.

Third, do you really care? If you don't drink fifteen cups of coffee a day, you are probably not going to learn anything useful related to the health effects of drinking coffee, no matter what the news. If you are a man or a postmenopausal woman, it doesn't matter how much mercury they found in your sushi—unless, of course, your daughter is planning on getting pregnant, in which case she has probably heard everything that's relevant from her obstetrician and does not need additional, unsubstantiated things to worry about from her parents.

Fourth, and most important, if you believe there may be news about an issue that concerns you and is worth the time exploring, spend the time it requires. Read the article in the newspaper, noting whether the purported outcome was simply an association observed in people followed over time or the definitive outcome of a randomized trial in which the outcome might legitimately be ascribed to the single intervention of interest (and was the only thing that differed between the participants). This may take a fair amount of medical literacy, particularly if you attempt to pursue the finding to its original source. This is rarely necessary. Any meaningful, important (and definitive) discovery will soon appear on reputable Websites. What are these? A sample list appears in the section on further reading. The best places to start are federal agencies, such as the Centers for Disease Control and Prevention, the National Institutes of Health, the Food and Drug Administration, the Agency for

Healthcare Research and Quality, and the Institute of Medicine (while not officially a federal agency, the IOM is congressionally chartered and fervently objective).

Other Web sources regularly contain helpful health information. Long-term coalitions offer legitimate expertise and research results; these include the American Heart Association, the American Cancer Society, and the Juvenile Diabetes Association (among others). Similarly, many professional societies (e.g., the American Academy of Pediatrics) closely follow relevant issues and are both reliable and current. Beware single-issue advocacy groups, as they inevitably have an agenda that is neither science-based nor objective. Their purpose is to raise an alarm (where sounder minds see no need) or look for adherents, advocates, or financial and political support. They almost never provide a balanced view.[4]

The Web has also sprouted potentially informative for-profit sites. Whether they make money from subscribers, catalogue sales, or marketing, it may be difficult to distinguish those that are comprehensively objective from those that are ill informed and meant to confound and confuse (often all three).

Want the bottom-line, most honest advice on healthy living? Don't smoke (that one is easy and backed by tons of data); drink alcohol but only in moderation (yes, most evidence suggests you'll live longer); get plenty of exercise; eat a balanced, low-salt, low-fat, low-calorie diet; and practice safe sex (assuming that remains on your agenda). If you want more specific advice, consult your physician. He or she will know about the latest drugs and tests worth knowing about; after all, physicians watch the same evening news that you do!

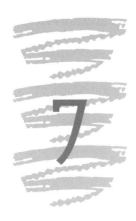

FROM SCIENCE TO POLICY
The Path Is Anything but Linear

Moving from data to policy (and practice) is a lot more complex and idiosyncratic than an outsider might suspect. I've outlined, in brief, the major steps (Figure 19). The process begins with scientific evidence. Sometimes, as is commonly the case for new drugs, the initial evidence is entirely unexpected.

RANDOM ACTS OF DISCOVERY
Aspirin was noted to retard the clotting of blood more than a century ago; it was tested (and proved modestly effective) for preventing heart attack less than forty years ago. As recently as a decade ago, the single factor that distinguished the higher quality of care a patient received for an acute heart attack at an academic medical center, when compared with a community hospital, was not sophisticated imaging or surgical facilities, but whether the patient was given aspirin on arrival.

Viagra, one of the best-known drugs in the world, was originally

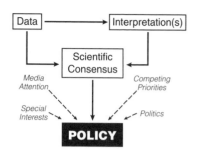

FIGURE 19. GOOD SCIENTIFIC DATA DO NOT NECESSARILY CHANGE HEALTH POLICY.
It usually takes forceful (and informed) advocacy to break through entrenched beliefs, background noise, distractions, and competing interests and priorities.

designed and tested to treat high blood pressure. Only when the trial failed and the participants were asked to return the unused pills did Viagra's real benefits surface: those in the control group dutifully returned their placebos; those given Viagra refused. The rest is history—except for one small but significant "health policy" footnote I'll return to below.

When men taking Proscar to slow the growth of their prostate found that they unexpectedly grew a bit of hair (more like peach fuzz), Merck had another runaway bestseller in Propecia, the same drug (finasteride), marketed at a much higher price, for balding. Many drugs discovered through laboratory research did what they were expected to do; nonetheless, it is remarkable how many were chance, unexpected (and highly profitable) revelations.

Hence the need for solid evidence with which to convince other scientists (and the Food and Drug Administration). Then, one needs to actually convince them. Basic laboratory scientists can readily test another scientist's observations. These laboratory replications usually suffice when the issue is a cellular receptor or a metabolic pathway.

Scientific consensus is often more elusive when the issue has clinical or health policy implications. New drugs and devices or surgical techniques can generally be subjected to randomized clinical trials, the ultimate "gold standard." But results can differ, depending on the selection of subjects, their stage or risk of disease, and a host of other variables. It sometimes takes numerous trials before a consensus is reached on both the benefits and the risks. Even when drugs are subjected to randomized trials, these never enroll sufficient numbers from every demographic group to provide solid proof for each group or any assurance about the real but infrequent risks once a drug begins to be used by millions of people.

One demographic regularly under-represented in drug trials is children. Drug makers (with the concurrence of the Food and Drug Administration) generally extrapolate the pediatric dose by age (and its rough association with plasma volume and body mass). But children are not just "small adults"; their organs work differently. Little provision is made for these differences, even when a sizable body of evidence suggests that the differences are important. Until someone "hollers"! Recently, as Baltimore's commissioner of health, Joshua Sharfstein (now the principal deputy commissioner of the FDA) organized his colleagues to "holler" about the high risks attendant to the use of over-the-counter cough and cold medicines marketed for children. The risks have proved high and the benefits nil, something a small group within the FDA already knew but were unable to convince senior policymakers to address. Less than a year after Sharfstein's group filed a formal (and highly publicized) petition for review, the FDA changed course; they've now pulled these drugs, for use by the youngest Americans, from the shelves.

As I previously suggested (Chapter 6), lots of important issues are simply not amenable to randomized trials. How could we determine what constitutes a balanced diet? We could randomly assign thousands (it might take millions) of people to eat alternative permutations and combinations of different foods, supplements, and beverages, and then wait years or centuries to witness the outcome. (It's more than likely that most of those enrolled in the trials wouldn't keep to their complicated and restricted choices.) We therefore rely instead on associations noted in observational studies and on common sense. Before a semblance of consensus can be

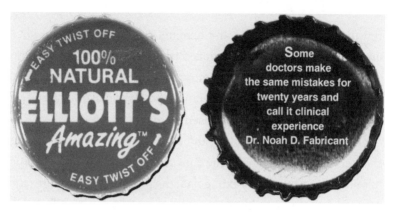

FIGURE 20. WISDOM CAN BE FOUND IN BOTTLE CAPS.
The outer and inner surfaces of a bottle cap from a beverage served at a working lunch. Who knew that beverage companies disseminated sophisticated medical insights? Source: Elliot's Amazing; photo by Alfred Sommer.

reached (if ever), these issues generally require multiple observational studies on different populations and from different perspectives, often augmented by experiments on laboratory animals.

For much the same reason (the overwhelming number of possible combinations and permutations of agents and interventions and ever-changing therapeutic options), most things we do in medicine have never been subjected to rigorous trials. Decisions are most often made on the basis of what we were taught in training, which itself was mostly based on clinical experience. One day I was offered bottled fruit juice during a meeting. To my astonishment, printed on the inside of the bottle's cap was: "Some doctors make the same mistakes for twenty years and call it clinical experience" (Figure 20). There's wisdom on the inside of bottle caps. It explains, in part, the wide variations in the way well-meaning physicians practice medicine (see Chapter 8).

When it comes to health policy, things get sticky. Advocacy by experts who know the evidence is important. But good scientists are rarely advocates, and most are readily outflanked by the belligerently ill informed. Early in my career, I joined two colleagues from the American Academy of Ophthalmology in testifying before Congress on the risks to health raised by then newfangled video display devices (e.g., what are now ubiquitous computer monitors). I subsequently spent nearly two years on a National Research Council committee reviewing the subject. Why all the fuss? Because one vocal "expert" insisted that these devices caused abortions, dermatological conditions, and a host of other dangerous side effects. When asked, under oath, whether I was certain this could never be the case, I responded, as a cautious and truthful scientist, "No, I can't be certain this can't ever occur." The strident advocate suffered no such inhibitions. And he was a "fellow scientist."[1]

When politics and "political" concerns enter the picture, policy and programs can suffer. Much of today's HIV epidemic in the United States is fueled by drug users sharing needles. One approach to reducing the spread of HIV is to provide users with clean needles. Will this stop drug use? No, but it will reduce the spread of HIV. Several carefully monitored studies have proved this. They have also proved that needle exchange (a new, clean needle for an old, dirty one) does not increase drug use. Here is an effective means of harm reduction. The Clinton White House agreed that the data were solid. Many in the public health community were surprised and deeply disappointed when the White House decided not to support needle-exchange efforts. The secretary of Health and Human Services readily admitted that the decision was entirely political.

Trumping judgment with politics is comparatively easy. The then-director of the National Cancer Institute (NCI) assembled an expert committee to review available evidence on mammography and recommend whether the age to initiate screening for breast cancer should be lowered from 50 years to 40. The committee, balancing the benefits of early detection against the increased risk of needless surgery triggered by false-positive results, recommended against it. The day the committee issued its report, NCI's director called the committee's recommendation "outrageous" (which makes you wonder why the NCI director formed the committee in the first place). At a congressional hearing that quickly followed, Senator Kay Hutchison exclaimed that "everyone in this room knows that by early detection we have saved lives" (what she failed to understand is that screening lots of women at age 40, when breast tissue is still dense, markedly reduces the chance of finding small tumors and markedly increases the risk of referring women without tumors for further work-up and needless biopsies). Dr. Donald Berry, chairman of biostatistics at M. D. Anderson Cancer Center, one of our country's foremost cancer treatment and research centers, pointed out that the benefits did not outweigh the risks, to which Senator Frist (formerly a cardiothoracic surgeon) "reminded everyone that Dr. Berry was a statistics expert and did not treat patients." If I ever needed an expert to balance scientific data, I'd want a respected biostatistician at my side.

You might as well know how it ended: the expert panel was fired and NCI recommended mammography at the earlier age.

Political posturing is not limited to the United States. Let's return to the Viagra story. Until Viagra came along, birth control pills had never been approved for use in Japan. For more than thirty years, the Japanese government had argued that Japanese women were different from Western women and might suffer untoward consequences from birth control drugs. But as soon as the FDA approved Viagra in the United States, the Japanese government approved Viagra's use by Japanese men. Japanese women were appropriately outraged; after decades of delay, the use of birth control pills was approved within months.

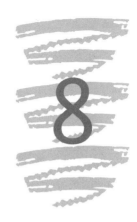

The U.S. Health Care System

The U.S. health care system is the subject of multivolume tomes. It is too complex and has too many moving parts for it to be described in any detail in a single chapter, much less to provide a prescription for its salvation. But some key aspects and core issues are worth pondering.

Calling U.S. medicine either "health care" or a "system" is an exaggeration. At its core, U.S. medicine is composed of individual physicians who are paid each time they treat a patient for a disease, mostly on a fee-for-service basis. They may work in solo practice or in small or large groups, but their organizational framework differs little from those of preindustrial craftsmen: they are paid for piecework.

This has important implications:

* Physicians are paid to treat our disease du jour, not to keep us healthy. "Health" has nothing to do with it (the most notable exception being pediatric "well-baby care").

* As treatments have become more complex and the knowledge needed more demanding, physicians have focused on narrower and narrower slices of disease; they "superspecialize." The piecework for which they get paid, never about health, is even less about optimizing outcomes for a sick person; the piecework is about treating a specific, limited slice of a sick person's disease(s).

* Any other "diseases" the patient might have are of little interest to the treating clinician because he or she does not have access to other physicians' records, doesn't have the time to inquire, and lacks the knowledge to make much sense of it, anyway.

* Nobody is coordinating our "care"; our most urgent illness receives all the attention. This poses enormous problems as we age and our litany of chronic diseases mounts: the treatment for some diseases makes others worse. In any case, who can keep track of all the medicines we are told to take (and who can afford them)?

* "Personalized medicine" was once the standard of practice. Physicians didn't just prescribe an antibiotic (during the heyday of personalized care, there were no antibiotics); the patient's "situation" (social, economic, cultural) was known and taken into account. There was no point in advising someone to get more rest and to relax if no one else was available to milk the cow or punch the timeclock. Today "personalized medicine" is invoked as a golden future awaiting genetic discoveries that will allow the pharmaceutical industry to create new drugs uniquely our own. Don't hold your breath![1]

Could physicians and other health care professionals be trained and incentivized to focus on keeping us healthy and coordinating our care? Of course, but for that we would need a real system, one that coordinated payments and training positions in a rational and objective manner, a system whose design (and financing) was constructed from whole cloth. U.S. medical care is underwritten by a multiplicity of financing schemes, each of which was developed at a unique moment in time. "In the beginning," patients paid a doctor directly for care (as some still do), which meant that only the wealthy received care. (Because physicians didn't have much of value to offer until relatively recently, this probably made little difference; the peasant and the merchant were equally likely to die from the plague.)

As medical care became more effective (and expensive), it came into greater demand. A variety of prepaid insurance plans, such as Blue Cross (for physicians' bills) and Blue Shield (for increasingly expensive hospital costs), were devised. The most radical formulation was Henry Kaiser's insurance scheme, in part because it provided both preventive and curative services but more because it was provided as a benefit of employment. This gambit was a competitive edge Kaiser used to recruit workers at a time when salaries were frozen by federally imposed wartime wage restraints. Employees pay no taxes on health benefits, though increasingly they are forgoing pay increases to maintain those benefits. Employer-based health coverage has since prevailed as the cornerstone of private American medical financing. In 1964 it was augmented by two additional schemes, Medicare and Medicaid, to pay the costs of caring for elderly people (age 65 or older) and those who were poor or disabled.

There we have it; the major (but by no means only) financial schemes that pay for our medical services. They differ from one another in how they are financed, what they cover, and how much

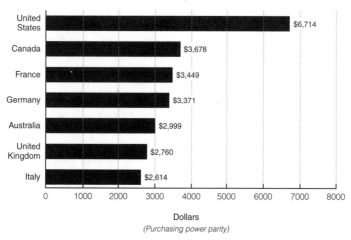

Health Care Spending
Per Capita - 2006

United States — $6,714
Canada — $3,678
France — $3,449
Germany — $3,371
Australia — $2,999
United Kingdom — $2,760
Italy — $2,614

Dollars
(Purchasing power parity)

FIGURE 21. WE SPEND A LOT ON HEALTH CARE.
Health care spending (in purchasing power parity) for selected market economies, 2006. The United States spent nearly twice as much on health care per person as our closest neighbor, Canada, and nearly three times as much as Italy or the United Kingdom. Source: Adapted from *Health Data*, 2008 (Organisation for Economic Co-operation and Development, 2007).

they pay. Each system has its own rules, and each seeks to contain its own costs.

If that's our "system," how much does it cost and what does it deliver? Unfortunately, "a lot" and "not nearly as much as it should," respectively.

As nearly everyone alive and literate knows (or should), the United States spends more on health care than any other nation on Earth. A lot more! In 2006 we spent $6,700 per person per year, twice (or more) what the United Kingdom, Canada, Germany, France, or Japan paid (Figure 21). That was more than 15 percent of our gross domestic product (GDP)—the total of all U.S. goods and services. The United Kingdom, Canada, Germany, France, and Japan spent between 8 and 11 percent of their GDP. And our health expenditures are growing rapidly. By 2007, the U.S. total surpassed $2 trillion (and 16 percent of our GDP).

In wealthy countries, health care spending is a "luxury," almost always increasing more quickly than overall GDP (or the typical "consumer price index"). This has been particularly the case for the profligate United States, where the increase in medical spending (in dollars) has greatly exceeded the overall growth in GDP or increase in inflation (Figures 22 and 23).

Surely, given how much we spend, we should receive the "best care available." Perhaps we do, but it is hard to know for sure. How does one measure the quality of a nation's health care system? Pre-

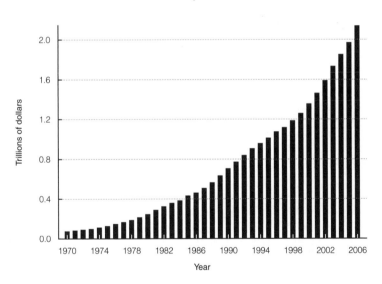

U.S. Health Expenditures in Dollars

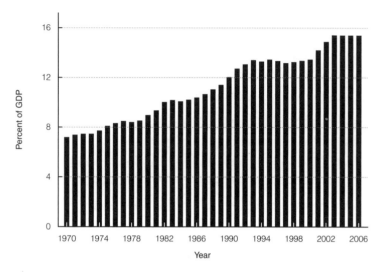

U.S. Health Expenditures as Percent of GDP

FIGURE 23. NEARLY EVERY YEAR HEALTH SPENDING IN THE
UNITED STATES ACCOUNTS FOR A LARGER SHARE
OF GROSS DOMESTIC PRODUCT.

U.S. health expenditure as a percentage of GDP, 1970–2006. The proportion of
U.S. GDP attributed to health care has doubled in the past two decades. Source:
Reprinted by permission from R. Pear, "Health Spending Exceeded Record $2 Trillion in
2006," New York Times, January 8, 2008.

sumably by the outcome: the health and longevity of its people. We
don't do well by those metrics. Americans certainly do not live longer than do citizens of other industrial nations; indeed, our life
expectancy at birth, 77 years, is about the same as Cuba's. Costa
Ricans live one year longer than we do, the French two years longer,
and the Japanese a full five years longer.[2]

As noted in Chapter 1, life expectancy is driven, to a large degree,
by infant mortality. Given our plethora of hospitals and neonatal
intensive care units, the United States must have exceedingly low
infant morality, right? Wrong! In 2006, thirty-two other countries
had lower infant mortality rates than the United States. We do bet-

ter on some other indices: among the twenty-five (of thirty) industrialized Organisation for Economic Co-operation and Development (OECD) countries that regularly report such data, ten had lower death rates from breast and prostate cancer and three had lower death rates from colon cancer. Good, to be sure, but not best.

Why aren't our health indices better? For a lot of reasons. Some arise from social and cultural issues, like high drug-use and homicide rates in our poor inner cities (the U.S. death rate from assault is an astounding six times the rate of all other OECD countries). Other reasons stem from the way we pay for and deliver medical care. In the latter category, our lack of universal health coverage looms large.

Why the United States, arguably the wealthiest large nation on Earth, fails to provide universal health care coverage must rank among the greatest mysteries to other nations. Among the thirty OECD countries (all of Western Europe and most of industrialized Asia and Latin America), only three lack universal health coverage: Turkey, Mexico, and the United States. It should be a source of national shame that we emulate Turkey and Mexico rather than the twenty-seven more advanced countries of the industrialized world. Our patchwork system, the marketing of competing (and confusing) plans, and the largely unregulated nature of care drive up costs and drive down outcomes.

Most revealing is that the costs of care and how medicine is practiced vary enormously across the United States; they even vary enormously across a single state. This is not necessarily because some doctors charge a great deal more than others; rather, it is because doctors practice medicine in different ways. This translates into more or less payment to doctors, but doctors' fees account for only about 20 percent of health care costs. More important, the manner in which doctors practice medicine affects the other 80 percent of those costs (MRI tests, CAT scans, surgical procedures, hospitalizations, drug prescriptions). Richard Lamm, former governor of Colorado, once joked that, to cut the costs of health care in the United States, we should borrow a trick from the agricultural sector. "Land banks" pay farmers to keep prime land idle; a "doctor bank" would pay doctors not to practice medicine! It would still cost us those doctors' salaries, but it would dramatically reduce the use of hospitals, tests, and interventions that account for the other 80 percent of health care costs!

Since that joke was made, we've discovered that we face a looming "doctor shortage." Part of that "shortage" is due to growing demand from the increased number of aged people in the population (and our accumulating chronic diseases), and part is due to the increased number of potentially beneficial tests and procedures to which we might "profitably" be subjected. But it is also related to where doctors like to live (in the same nice places that everyone else likes) and how doctors like to practice (caring for conditions that don't require night-call and receiving the most lucrative reimbursement).

We face a growing paradox: highly qualified physicians complain that they don't have enough patients, largely because they live in the same places as similarly minded colleagues, while great numbers of Americans live in communities virtually bereft of medical services (think rural America and impoverished inner-city communities). Poor areas of Harlem, Detroit, Philadelphia, and Baltimore desperately need doctors. But large variations in the concentration of physicians ensure that some doctors will have relatively fewer patients than they would like, while those few physicians working in difficult locales, in which reimbursement rates are much lower, are overwhelmed with work.

By 2030, according to some estimates, the United States will need to import as many as 200,000 physicians to meet our growing demands. Where will they come from? Poor countries, which can least afford to lose them. Something is wrong with this picture! The wealthiest nation on Earth is not training sufficient physicians for its needs so, instead, it steals them from countries that need them more.

We can begin to solve our self-inflicted problems in many ways. We could start by giving teeth to a system feebly implemented decades ago: vary physician remuneration in ways that better serve society. Pay more to those who work in underserved areas and less to those who live where they are least needed. A similar system could help rebalance young physicians' choices of specialty: comprehensive care for elderly people might be reimbursed at the same level as interventionist care for heart attacks and strokes.

It is unlikely that our health care system can be seriously fixed "one piece at a time." The solutions require a "systems approach." But, the United States being what it is, progress is likely to be slow and incremental, bandages applied at the periphery of an increasingly dysfunctional patchwork of health care activities.

One (but only one) of the reasons many medical students choose to become "interventionists" instead of family physicians is that the cost of medical education has left them highly indebted. The average medical student graduates with $140,000 of debt, largely lent at commercial interest rates. With another three to eight years of training at apprentice wages, highly paid subspecialties are the surest way to support a family and pay off accumulated debt. One could mitigate this issue in any number of ways: pay higher subsidies for medical training (while varying subsidies in ways that address underserved populations and specialties); raise reimbursement rates differentially to accomplish the same socially beneficial end; and redefine which tasks and roles require the education and skills of a fully trained physician and which can be delegated, just as effectively and a lot more efficiently, to specially trained nonphysicians (nurse-practitioners and physician assistants). We have an even greater shortage of nurses than of physicians—but for different reasons.

The exploitation of some resident trainees, who now fill slots in underserved areas, needs as much a mandate as a carrot. Just before stepping down from the Senate, Patrick Moynihan cornered a huge piece of pork for New York City. Its largest teaching hospitals agreed to reduce the number of specialists they trained in exchange for a payment of $400 million by the federal government (officialdom was worried that too many physicians were being trained; in reality, too many were being trained who wanted to live in the same place and practice the same specialties). At the end of the first year, the hospitals returned the money. It was too expensive to incentivize fully trained practitioners to do the jobs that hospitals were able to delegate to (generally foreign-educated) medical trainees. There is something wrong with a several trillion dollar "system" that can't solve so direct a challenge.

Whatever is true for physicians is equally true for other health professionals. Nurses are in short supply; they work long hours that are disruptive to family life, for little pay, in far more intensive and stressful work environments than ever before. Working conditions and reimbursement are fixable items in a systems sense; far less so if each profession, institution, and organization must fend (and find solutions) for itself.

Can we seriously change what we pay for without increasing overall spending? Might there be enough elasticity in the overall costs of U.S. health care to allow for modest realignments? Absolutely! All we lack is imagination and political will.

The cost of medical care varies tremendously across the United States. Need evidence? In 2003, Medicare spent an average of $5,400 per enrollee living in Minneapolis and $11,500 per enrollee living in Miami. That's a big difference! Because no one claims that seniors in Minneapolis are any less healthy than are seniors in Miami, the celebrated Princeton health economist and critic Uwe Reinhardt asked provocatively: "How can it be that the 'best medical care in the world' costs twice as much as the 'best medical care in the world'?" Because a lot of that care isn't necessary!

Where does the extra funding go in high-cost areas? In part, it pays for extra days in the hospital (and extra days in the ICU) during the last months of life. There is no evidence that these extra investments improve patient satisfaction or medical outcome.

Some of the variation in medical costs is related to patient expectations, but the largest part is related to what doctors ultimately do (and prescribe). Perfectly competent, intelligent, and well-meaning physicians practice medicine differently. Jack Wennberg first hit on this phenomenon in the 1960s and has chronicled it ever since. Early on, he compared the rates at which physicians in the relatively small state of Rhode Island treated patients with exactly the same conditions. It turned out that some physicians recommended (and performed) tonsillectomies 15 times as often as others, not because their patients had more sore throats but because that was what many had been trained to do, decades before. Others performed radical mastectomies (for breast cancer) 50 times more frequently, prostatectomies 15 times more frequently, and disc excisions 30 times more frequently than colleagues a few miles away. Surely all these (different) rates couldn't have been the "right" rates. Some must have been too low and some too high.

These "small area variations" helped convince medical leaders of the need to provide guidance on what the "right" indications for various interventions, and therefore the right rates, ought to be. By employing more and better evidence and converting these into practical "clinical guidelines," most specialties have begun to reduce needless variation, raise standards, and improve the quality of care. Practice guidelines could ultimately save a great deal of money as well, funds that could be better deployed in support of needed "systems change." As the great English statistician William Farr recognized back in 1837, "medical science [and clinical practice] will advance not by . . . opinions and assertions but by registering facts . . . by applying that mighty instrument of natural science—arithmetic."[3]

One of the major factors driving rates of intervention (and associated medical costs) is the concentration of physicians and hospital beds. Communities with more surgeons experience more surgery; communities with more hospital beds experience more frequent hospitalization. New Haven had only half the number of hospital beds as Boston; the population of New Haven was hospitalized only half as often as were Bostonians—without any evidence that Connecticut Yankees suffered from medical neglect. More stringent reimbursement standards have begun to bring hospital admission rates (among well-served communities) into greater alignment. But those states with higher Medicare expenditures also had more medical specialists and fewer general practitioners.

Another factor driving interventions and costs is misplaced incentives. Our (largely) fee-for-service reimbursement scheme pays for "disease-work." Capitation is an alternative model for financing and delivering care: physicians (and institutions) are paid a flat fee to maintain the health of their pool of patients. Done properly, with sufficient resources and ingenuity, capitation can drive important health care priorities unrelated to costs alone. As an ophthalmologist, I was routinely graded on the quality of my cataract and glaucoma surgery; that is, on my technical skill. Was my surgery effective? Was my rate of complications low? It did not matter that some patients who needed my attention were never referred for care or were not referred until late in the course of their glaucoma, when there was little I could do for them.

In a well-run capitation scheme, the health plan is responsible for the health of its members. Its grade depends as much on glaucoma patients being recognized and receiving the attention they deserve as it does on the technical quality with which that care is delivered. In other words, the grade depends on the infrequency with which members enrolled in the plan go blind from glaucoma. This is a far more powerful perspective—and score card. What is important is that my team won the World Series, not that I had a uniquely outstanding batting average. In general, patients fare better in a system judged on everyone's outcome; such a system can also save costs by changing basic incentives. In 1997, a group of ophthalmologists in Saint Louis switched from a traditional fee-for-service system to capitated care. The number of cataract operations fell by more than half, without any evidence that those who needed cataract surgery were denied it (Figure 24).

Several health maintenance organizations (HMOs), such as Kaiser-Permanente, offer outstanding capitated care. It makes sense for them to coordinate the care of all their patients' ills and to provide preventive services that keep people healthy in the first place. Most private health insurance plans refuse to spend money on prevention or on anything else that will make people healthier and their future care less costly (including routine, periodic screening for glaucoma; prostate, colon, and breast cancer; and the like). They reason that enrollees switch health plans every three years. They don't consider it in their economic interest to pay to prevent a disease (and its attendant medical care and costs) that won't occur until the person is in some other plan, where the savings will be realized. But if all plans were mandated to provide similarly effective preventive services, they would all benefit financially downstream, regardless of which plan a patient happened to be in at the moment the disease didn't occur!

A lot of unnecessary medical costs arise from the adoption of inappropriate technology. One glaring example will serve for many.

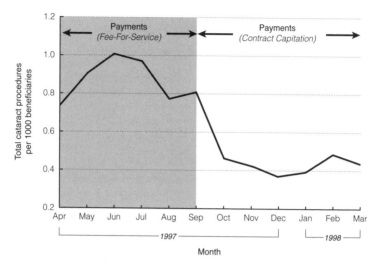

FIGURE 24. IF YOU PAY FOR PIECEWORK, YOU GET MORE PIECEWORK.
Change in cataract surgical rates in the Barnes Eye Care Network when they
changed their reimbursement system from fee-for-service to contracted capitation. Under fee-for-service, ophthalmologists were paid (rewarded) each time they
performed a cataract operation. The more operations they performed, the more
they were paid. When the payment scheme switched to a capitation system, in
which income was not related to the number of operations performed, cataract
surgical rates fell by half. Source: Reprinted by permission from W. Shrank, S. L. Ettner,
P. H. Slavin, et al., "Effect of Physician Reimbursement Methodology on the Rate and Cost
of Cataract Surgery," *Archives of Ophthalmology* 123 (2005): 1736, Figure 2. Copyright © 2005
American Medical Association. All rights reserved.

Between 1960 and 1980, the rate of cesarean sections in the United
States rose from 6 percent of all deliveries to 24 percent (Figure 25).
Most of that rise is attributed to the introduction of electronic fetal
monitors, instruments attached to women in labor that sound an
alarm when they register evidence of fetal distress (primarily
changes in the fetus's heart rate). This might seem like a good thing,
as it apparently was. The alarm goes off, the mother is wheeled into
the operating room, and the baby is quickly delivered by C-section

before suffering irreversible harm. While it seemed to make sense (like so much new gadgetry inevitably does), there is little evidence that it makes a difference! There have been more than a dozen trials comparing electronic fetal monitoring to old-fashioned auscultation (listening to the fetal heart through a stethoscope placed on the mother's abdomen). Fetal monitoring did not improve fetal outcomes; all it did was raise the number of (uninterpretable) alarms and, as a consequence, the number of cesarean sections.

Professional societies have striven, with only modest success, to

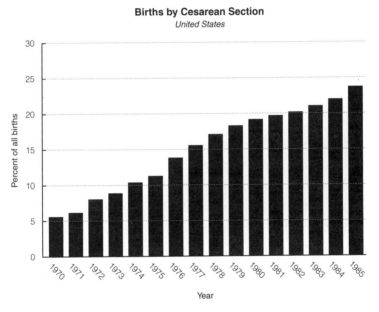

Births by Cesarean Section
United States

FIGURE 25. UNPROVEN TECHNOLOGY OFTEN DRIVES CLINICAL PRACTICE.
Births by cesarean section in the United States, 1970–1985. The growing use of fetal monitors, which signal potential fetal distress, led to a marked increase in the number of babies delivered by cesarean section. Source: Data from a series of reports in the Centers for Disease Control and Prevention's Morbidity and Mortality Weekly Report. Summary data available at "Rates of Cesarean Delivery, United States, 1993," MMWR 44, no. 15 (April 21, 1995): 303–7.

reduce the rate of unnecessary C-sections. The use of fetal monitors is now so widespread and the fear of litigation if a nonmonitored child is born with a neurological deficit (as some always will be, monitor or not) that the use of monitors (and the high rate of C-sections) has been little affected. In Brazil, nearly half of all children born in the public sector are delivered by C-section; in the private sector, the rate is more than 80 percent.

Among the many absurd ways in which we attempt to improve the care that Americans receive, perhaps the most absurd of all is how little we spend on studies to ensure it. The National Institutes of Health (NIH) spends more than $30 billion every year, much of it on basic laboratory research to discover new genes and processes that might better explain disease and spur the development of new preventive measures and treatments. The rest is spent on clinical trials to determine whether new tests, drugs, and procedures have value (most drug trials are financed by the pharmaceutical company in a position to profit from the drug's approval and subsequent sales). The Agency for Healthcare Research and Quality, charged with identifying appropriate treatments people should receive and the degree to which they receive them, is provided a measly $350 million a year, or 1 cent for each NIH dollar. Why bother supporting the discovery of new genes and drugs if we don't also determine which drugs work best and under what circumstances and whether or not Americans are receiving the most appropriate treatment?

We are often told that the United States can't afford universal health insurance. If that were true, how would Canada, Germany, Switzerland, France, Spain, Italy, and the United Kingdom afford it? We are also often told, by way of obfuscation, that countries with "universal coverage" have long waiting lists for care and that, when Canadians are really sick, they flee south, to the United States, for their care. This is rubbish! I've yet to see data documenting that large numbers of sick Canadians clog our border crossings, and none whatsoever to indicate that Canadians would trade their health care system for ours. Canadians, Japanese, Germans, Spaniards, and British all receive urgent, life-saving care when they need it. What they don't necessarily receive, unless they are willing to pay for it in the private sector or in another country, is all the care they want whenever they want it. Countries like Canada and the United Kingdom, which limit health care expenditures, have waiting lists for nonurgent interventions (such as cataract removal and hip replacement).

Wealthy patients might elect to come to the United States and pay to receive care immediately, instead of waiting in a queue for care that is "rationed" at home. But this is less a reflection on the effectiveness of universal coverage than it is on the amount of money a country is willing to spend on health care. While the United States spends more than 15 percent of its GDP on health care, Canada spends less than 10 percent. Canada could rid itself of waiting lists by simply raising spending to 12 percent of its GDP. Without abandoning universal coverage, it would still underspend the United States. Because it spends less, Canada performs fewer expensive tests and procedures but without necessarily impairing outcomes. A 1997 study showed that Americans who had a heart attack were six times more likely to receive angioplasty or bypass surgery than were Canadians, with no apparent difference in survival (Figure 26). Americans intuitively understand that there is a monumental problem with our costs of care. Nearly two-thirds consider "poultry" and "video rentals" to be good value for their money; fewer than a fifth feel the same about hospital charges (Figure 27).

The fact is, every nation rations care. Most do so explicitly. The English decide, through ongoing, spirited political exchanges, how much they are willing to spend on medical care and use the rest on other public goods, such as roads and schooling. Having set the

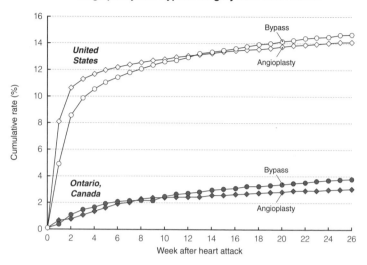

Angioplasty and Bypass Surgery after Heart Attack

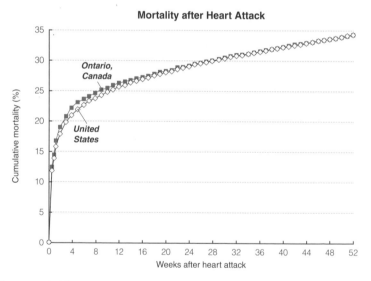

Mortality after Heart Attack

FIGURE 26. MORE CLINICAL INTERVENTION DOES NOT NECESSARILY
IMPROVE CLINICAL OUTCOME.

The rates of coronary angioplasty and bypass surgery performed on patients with
heart attacks in the United States and Ontario, Canada (top), and their death rates
over the ensuing year (bottom). Despite far higher rates of surgery in the United
States, mortality in the two areas was identical. Source: Reprinted by permission from

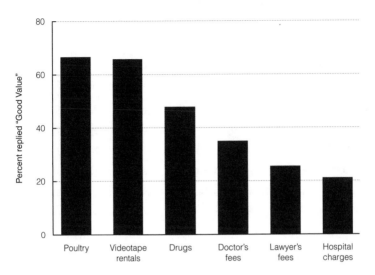

Public Views on the "Value for Cost"

Percent replied "Good Value"

Poultry — Videotape rentals — Drugs — Doctor's fees — Lawyer's fees — Hospital charges

amount for medical care, they then agree on what will be paid for and what won't. As Enoch Powell, former U.K. minister of health, observed, "There is virtually no limit to the amount of health care an individual is capable of absorbing."[4] The accepted standards of care and the investments needed to support them change with the times (and with political pressure).

Thus were "rationing" and "waiting lists" born. In the United Kingdom, the wealthy can still go outside the system for care that society is not willing to provide (in sufficient numbers or with sufficient alacrity) from the public till. Because public spending is sensitive to political processes, the amount spent on health care is increased whenever rationing becomes tighter and waiting lists become longer than society is willing to accept.

The United States also rations care, but we do so implicitly: if you can afford care, you receive it; if you can't, you don't. Those of us fortunate to have generous health insurance largely get what we need. A lot of what we've decided we need, however, is not essential; it is convenient, lifestyle-enhancing, or whatever the pharmaceutical industry has convinced us we can't live without (a purple pill?). But most health care plans no longer pay for the frivolous; increasingly, they won't pay for the latest, most expensive drug either, unless it truly makes a difference.

MARKET FORCES: GOOD FOR ECONOMISTS BUT NOT FOR PATIENTS

There is little question that we can reduce our health care costs because there is no compelling reason why we need to spend so much more than the rest of the industrialized world. But, being the United States, we've decided the way to do this is to employ market forces rather than informed judgment or social discourse. Rational pocketbook discipline can help—at the margins. Increasingly, health plans make us pay more for brand name drugs when there are generic versions that are just as good (and a lot cheaper).

But the public is in no position to make informed choices when it comes to "big-ticket" items. Indulge me with this analogy:

> Over drinks one evening, I tell you about my fantastic new virtual-reality home entertainment center. I can not only watch an Orioles game but also pitch it. I predict that you will ask me two questions (what I can't predict is the order in which you will ask them): "Where

did you get it?" and "How much did it cost?" My answer: "Oh, about $5 million." To which you would probably respond, "I'll wait until the price comes down."

Now let's imagine that you are in the emergency room and the physician tells you that your daughter needs life support and a hugely complicated emergency procedure to try to correct a bleeding aneurysm in her brain. You do not ask, "How much does it cost?" nor do you ask "Where can I get it cheaper?" You don't even care if the chance of success is less than 10 percent. You want it done now, and you want it done by whoever is the best in the world. (Of course, you have no idea how to find out who is the best in the world.)

No economist can claim, with a straight face, that a patient in need of critical care (and most care is critical to the patient who needs it) is in a position to hunt for the most cost-effective version. Patients don't know enough about the vagaries of care to begin to ask the right economic questions or make economically appropriate decisions; what's more, they are too anxious to care. They naturally want only one thing: that they (or their loved one) receive the best care available.

Parts of our health care system do respond "rationally" to market forces, often to the detriment of society. Insurance companies are a prime example. Like any business, an insurance company's main aim is to maximize profits. If publicly owned, the company is legally mandated to maximize shareholder value, which is generally interpreted as much the same thing. How do the companies lawfully do this? By minimizing costs (the amount of care they pay for) and maximizing income (charging the highest rates—or imposing the largest deductibles—that the market will bear). How does this work in practice? Among other stratagems, insurance companies try not to enroll anyone who might get sick! This includes individuals who have less-than-stellar family histories, who are over a certain age, or who belong to a particularly high-care racial, economic, or social demographic group.

And individuals and small businesses—it is not worth their risk of a single catastrophic illness whose costs they can't spread across a large group of other enrollees who don't get sick. When my son, then a healthy, 35-year-old lawyer, decided to begin a Web start-up, my wife and I insisted that he buy top-quality health insurance, the kind we had. We were dismayed to discover that the cost ran more than twelve thousand dollars a year—for a single, young, HIV-negative professional! Small businesses face the same problem. If a single employee develops an expensive illness, whether renal failure, cancer, or AIDS, the employer's premium the next year will skyrocket (assuming the policy isn't dropped altogether).

Spurring competition between health care plans is a sorry way to attempt to contain costs. The theory is that Americans will choose the most cost-effective plan. But Americans are in no position to figure out which is the most cost-effective, and who wants the most cost-effective plan in the first place? What most of us want is a plan that will provide high-quality care when we need it, without driving us into bankruptcy.

For those fortunate enough to have a choice of health care plans, making a fully informed decision about which to choose it is nearly impossible, in part because different plans structure their options, co-pays, deductibles, and a host of other variables differently (purposely or not).

One personal example: for nearly thirty years, my employer, the Johns Hopkins University, has offered me a choice of health plans. They vary in cost and coverage. Because I am reasonably well compensated and cautious by nature, I always chose the top Blue Cross/Blue Shield plan. For years it had been the most expensive option, but the subsidized cost of the premium was less than the "benefit dollars" I was allotted until about fifteen years ago, when I was surprised to discover that the cost of the plan now exceeded my "benefits." Choosing the top plan would cost me additional dollars, out of pocket. As best I could tell, the "real" cost of the top plan was $4,800; the BC/BS plan one step below mine cost only $945. These must be two very different plans! As a reasonably informed health care strategist, I delved into the fine print. I was not really interested in co-pays and deductibles, which varied considerably between the two plans. What interested me was the bottom line: if my and my wife's health went to hell in a basket, what was the most that the care could cost me? To my surprise (and disbelief), both plans appeared to cap my costs at $2,000!

Clearly, I did not understand the differences between these two plans. How could one plan cost $4,000 more than the other, when the expenses both might entail, in a worst-case scenario, were only half that?

The Benefits Office at Johns Hopkins could not provide an explanation and suggested I call Blue Cross/Blue Shield directly. After a week pondering the problem, Blue Cross/Blue Shield found the answer: the plans were "experience rated." That meant that the premium charged those in the top plan was determined by the costs of caring for those in the top plan. Who enrolled in the top plan? People who were elderly or sick or at high risk of becoming sick. Their cost of care was high; hence, their premiums were high. Those who enrolled in the cheaper plan were younger and healthier and chose the "cheaper" plan because they did not expect to need expensive care.

Both groups seemingly made a "rational" market decision, one that economists might applaud. But those who purchased the top plan did so on a faulty premise—that if it cost more, it must provide better coverage. It took careful digging and a lot of wasted time for me, someone with more than a passing acquaintance with the health care system, to identify the appropriate choice: the cheaper plan. From an "insurance" perspective, it was just as generous as the far more expensive plan at far lower cost. How is the average American, without my background and interest (and, perhaps, with more urgent things to attend to) supposed to navigate these waters?

For whom else do market forces work? For physicians, pharmaceutical companies, the makers of medical devices, hospitals, nursing homes, pharmacists, and the like. They want to maximize revenues and minimize costs. They have the luxury of time, expertise, and multiple business plans from which thoughtfully to choose. A study published in the Journal of the American Academy of Dermatology revealed that patients had to wait twenty-six days to have a potentially malignant mole examined but only eight days if they wanted Botox injections to smooth out their wrinkles. With the proliferation of cosmetic interventions, dermatologists now make more than twice as much as internists and pediatricians—more, in fact, than general surgeons![5]

"Big Pharma" is all about profits. And they'll charge whatever the market will bear. When their drug is unique—and uniquely effective—the sky's the limit. A drug's price depends entirely on its anticipated demand. Unlike bread or even automobiles, it has little to do with the cost of production. Genzyme, for example, has a unique drug, Cerezyme, for the treatment of the rare but debilitating entity, Gaucher disease. Its drug generates more than $1 billion in revenue annually. How can a drug used by fewer than five thousand patients generate that much revenue? By charging $300,000 for a year's supply!

Genentech developed a pioneering drug, Avastin, originally approved for the treatment of metastatic colon cancer. One dose, an intravenous injection of 4 ml or more, was priced at $1,000 to $2,000. Genentech then reformulated the same active agent in a way they claimed would make it more effective for the treatment of macular degeneration, and named it Lucentis. One dose of Lucentis, an intraocular injection of only 0.05 ml, was priced—you guessed it—at $2,000.

Only the patient—society at large—is incapable of responding "rationally" to the health care "market."

Market forces are not the best basis on which to build a great health care system! Other countries are as befuddled as we are by their inability to slow the growth in health care costs and even occasionally look to our experiences for direction. But they have not abandoned their traditional systems. While no population is entirely satisfied with its health care system, Americans are a lot less satisfied than most (Figure 28). A 2008 Harris Interactive poll found that

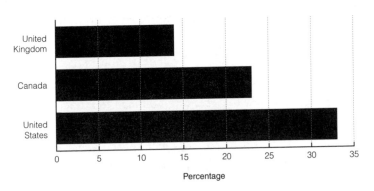

**Percentage of Public Who Said Their
Health Care System Needed to Be Rebuilt**

FIGURE 28. NEED ONE SAY MORE?
Percentage of the public in the United Kingdom, Canada, and the United States who said their health care system needed to be rebuilt from scratch. These three comparable English-speaking countries have different systems for organizing and paying for health care. Fully one-third of Americans, a proportion more than twice as high as in the United Kingdom, said their system needed to be completely rebuilt. Source: Data from K. Donelan, R. J. Blendon, C. Schoen, et al., "The Cost of Health System Change: Public Discontent in Five Nations," Health Affairs 18 (1999): 206–16.

33 percent of Americans but only 15 percent of Brits thought that their health care system needed to be completely rebuilt.

Meanwhile, Americans without insurance (the self-employed, unemployed, underemployed, and those working for small businesses or for large businesses at minimum wage) receive too little care, which is often delayed and almost always more expensive than it needs to be. They also suffer the health consequences. A recent study found that, when those without insurance reached 65 and became eligible for Medicare, their use of services and their health indices improved dramatically.[6]

The poor are less healthy than the rest of us (see Chapter 9), for a lot of reasons—some cultural, some economic, and some related to their inability to access timely health care. Medicaid, and now SCHIP (State Children's Health Insurance Program), are meant to address some of these impediments by paying for critical services needed by mothers and their children. Most men younger than 65 are left "out in the cold." But it is not easy for even mothers and children to access care.

Medicaid, supported jointly by federal and state funding, is chronically underfinanced. As a result, reimbursement rates are extremely low—so low that it is often difficult to attract physicians to practice in areas where Medicaid is widely used or to accept Medicaid beneficiaries as patients. For several years, Maryland's Eastern Shore lacked a single obstetrician willing to provide services to Medicaid patients; obstetricians claimed that the reimbursement did not cover even the cost of malpractice insurance.

Simply having practitioners willing to accept Medicaid does not necessarily overcome all the obstacles to medical access. Baltimore has a terrible public transportation system. Simply to obtain well-baby care and its attendant immunizations, a single mother sometimes needs to visit several locations, in different parts of town, necessitating her missing a full day's work. Enough such days can cost her her job.

Emergency rooms are everyone's medical care fallback. Those with little regular access to health services routinely rely on emergency rooms. But this is neither efficient nor effective, and it presents major problems for the rest of us.

Emergency rooms are for emergencies; I don't want the ER to be clogged up with patients with routine illnesses when I am having a stroke or heart attack or when my son or daughter has been in an auto accident. ERs are also extremely expensive. They are packed with costly equipment and specialized personnel. These costs need to be covered, whether the patient needs them or not. An average "visit" to an ER might cost a hospital $450; a typical well-baby visit in the clinic costs $75.

ERs are not a place anyone should need for routine care. ERs are, by necessity, focused on brief, urgent, life-saving interventions. The staff, procedures, and mind-set are entirely unsuited for routine illnesses, long-term oversight of an infant's development, or the coordination of care for an elderly person's multiple chronic illnesses. Upset stomachs, back pains (some of which might herald a deadly condition), "flu," and mothers with feverish babies by necessity are left to sit out the night.

By the time many people get to an emergency room for a "routine" illness, they need more care than they otherwise would have needed. Those who lack insurance are likely to delay seeking care until their illness is more severe, and they are not likely to receive valuable preventive services. In the 1970s, when care was a lot less costly than it is today, the Rand Corporation carried out a massive experiment on health insurance. People were randomly allocated to different levels of coverage, with different co-pays and deductibles. Not surprisingly, those with the highest level of coverage and the lowest co-pay sought the most care. Little, if any, of that care was inappropriate. In contrast, those without coverage (or with other strong financial disincentives from seeking care) sought less care—until, that is, they were sicker and required more intensive (and expensive) care.

A recent study of Medicare "managed care" plans found that even small co-payments (ten to twenty dollars) significantly reduced breast cancer screening (mammography) among women who should have received it, regardless of their income or ethnicity. Those who were African American or who came from poorer and less well-educated communities were doubly disadvantaged because they were more likely to have enrolled in plans requiring co-payments!

Enlightened corporations are discovering that economic disincentives to seeking care and filling prescriptions can hurt the corporation's own bottom line. By reducing co-payments required for asthma medications, Pitney-Bowes reduced the annual costs of caring for asthma among its beneficiaries by 15 percent. "Market forces" do indeed work, to the disadvantage of those who can't afford health insurance (or additional out-of-pocket expenses).

Not everyone who lacks health insurance is poor. Some find the cost prohibitive despite a middle-class income because of the higher premiums charged the self-employed and those working for small businesses. Even those who can afford to pay individual premiums sometimes choose not to. A disproportionate number are young and healthy. Why pay for insurance when you have little reason to believe that you may get sick? If you do contract some dreadful illness (say, renal failure requiring life-long dialysis or a kidney transplant), the costs will far exceed your means. You will go bankrupt, and the rest of us will end up paying the costs of your care. This is neither fair nor appropriate.[7]

Health insurance is like life insurance, auto insurance, and fire insurance: you hope not to collect, but if you need to, you're covered. Just like fire insurance, health insurance must spread the costs as widely as possible; among those who will need care and those who won't (without knowing precisely who those will be beforehand). That reduces the average cost of insurance, making it more affordable (and equitable). This is why everyone needs to be "in the system," not just those who are sick or who think they might get sick.

The rest of the modern world considers (appropriate) health care a "right." We accept this principle in other spheres: every child has the right to attend school; fire departments fight all fires, not just fires in the homes of the wealthy; the police (more or less) protect everyone from violent crime. Why are we willing to pay for these public services? Because they enrich us all; they make us a better, wealthier, more secure, and productive nation. But they also make sense (and cents). Crime that strikes the person walking beside me endangers me as well; if my neighbor's house is on fire, my house is at risk of going up in flames; and public schools and colleges ensure that the United States has the educated work force our modern economy requires. By the same token, if my waiter, co-worker, or laundress has multiple-drug-resistant tuberculosis and is not receiving appropriate care, my risk of becoming infected is greatly increased. Health care is a public good; everyone benefits when everyone else receives the care that he or she needs.

Can we afford to provide everyone with essential care? To a significant degree, we already do. Taxpayers already cover the health care costs of elderly (Medicare) patients, many of the poor and disabled (Medicare, Medicaid, and SCHIP), veterans, federal, state, county, and city employees, those with AIDS, and the like. These publicly financed programs cover more than half of all health care expenditures in the United States, considerably more than is financed by traditional, private health insurance. Add to these the costs of uncompensated care—the care provided to those who never pay. The rest of us ultimately cover those costs through federal subsidies and higher insurance premiums and hospital charges. Finally, those of us receiving insurance as a "benefit" of employment are actually paying for our insurance in the form of lower wages. Add it all together and the real costs for universal coverage can't be very different from what we now pay in multiple, varied, opaque, and disjointed ways.

Adopting universal coverage through a transparent system could prove cheaper (though I wouldn't wager on that). One of the reasons other nations can invest less in health and have better outcomes is that they waste less on administrative overhead. Canadians spend only four cents of every health care dollar on overhead; Medicare does almost as well, at six cents. But when private insurance companies attempted to "manage" our care—a euphemism for managing their "costs"—they spent more than thirty cents of every dollar on approval (and denial) processes, marketing, and profits. Now that they do less "managing" of care, they get by on a bit less "overhead."

Some analysts estimate that our overuse of medical products and procedures accounts for another 20 percent of excess costs. Simply reducing overhead and minimizing the use of unnecessary drugs and procedures (by excluding them from the essential package of care) should cover the costs of insuring the 15 percent of Americans who are presently uninsured. This is obviously a rough, ballpark figure, but it indicates that we can get by on a lot less spending and use the difference to cover much of the cost of universal care. The rest of the industrialized world already does.

Providing universal coverage should not prove difficult, but containing the growth in health care costs will. As populations grow and age, the amount of illness needing care increases. (As is often pointed out, as much as one-third of all health care cost is incurred during the last three months of life. This is not a particularly practical insight because we don't often know which those last three months are!)

Every country is concerned about the rapid escalation in health care costs. The Kaiser Family Foundation estimates that the cost of employer-sponsored health plans rose by nearly 80 percent over the past five years.[8] While no one knows how high health care spending can go without wrecking our economy, we do know that the cost of health care is already diverting resources from other social programs (education, housing, parks, transportation). All new drugs, devices, and surgical procedures add to those costs, while few of these innovations offer dramatic benefits over existing technology. The populations of most countries undergo long, intense debate to reach societal agreement on just how much should be spent, and on what.

The United States would obviously benefit from a fresh, new look at how we deliver and pay for care and from a willingness to consider radical reforms for more efficient and effective delivery and financing systems. But such openness is not likely. Too many powerful players have too much at stake, and too many Americans fear that they may end up with less than they currently have.

The costs are growing too large and too fast, and this growth worries states (who pay benefits and co-fund Medicaid) and the federal government (which pays for Medicare and much of Medicaid). Most potently, perhaps, rising health care costs are making U.S. businesses less competitive in the globalized economy—they must first recoup the costs of providing health care to their aging workers (and, in some instances, their retirees) before they can even begin to compete with foreign industries on productivity. It is now widely known that the U.S. auto industry spends more on health care costs than on steel: twenty-five hundred dollars per vehicle, which goes straight to the sticker price (or is deducted from the bottom line).

A reformed U.S. health care system would ideally have the following attributes:

* Every American must have basic health care coverage (however that might ultimately be defined).

* Those who can pay for insurance will pay for it (whether through taxes or other means); those who can't pay will have their premiums subsidized (to the degree required by their incomes).

* The costs of essential care for all Americans must be equitably distributed across all Americans. This does not mean that health care providers need to be government employees, but it does mean that everyone needs to be in the "pool," sick and well alike. A "single payer" for care (and a single entity that equitably spreads the costs and collects the funds needed to cover those costs) is the simplest way to achieve this. This, essentially, is the way Medicare works.

* Americans need to agree, through thoughtful and informed debate, on what constitutes a "basic health care package." The calculus will include the cost-effectiveness of competing drugs and procedures and, importantly, on what conditions, in which age groups, our funds will be spent. The basic health care package needs to reflect what our society values most. When Oregon launched its original Medicaid reforms, it established a total budget for the program and then listed the conditions, in order of priority, deserving treatment. The line between what would be funded and what wouldn't was drawn at the point where funds ran out. The initial list ranked interventions on the basis of their "cost-benefit." "Capping teeth" had a higher cost-benefit than treating childhood leukemia; initially, capping teeth was above the line and treating

leukemia was below. But the public decided that treating a life-threatening disease in children trumped a mostly cosmetic procedure. Priority for treating the two conditions was reversed. That's why political discourse needs to determine not only how much will be spent but also on what it will be spent.

* Those with the means should be permitted to purchase additional insurance to cover conditions outside the basic package. These additional insurance packages need to be offered in standard, readily understood increments, so that the public can compare competing plans rather than being befuddled by them. The differences in coverage provided by level A, level B, and level C plans should be clear and precisely the same across all insurance providers. These supplemental insurance plans would compete on the level of service they provide and the prices they charge. The purchasing public could then knowledgeably choose among different insurance companies; the most efficient, service-oriented companies willing to make the smallest profits would prevail.

* The U.S. government (or its agent) must aggressively negotiate the lowest appropriate price for drugs and devices. Nongeneric prescription drugs cost 20 to 50 percent more in the United States than in Canada and sometimes 100 percent more than in Italy. An uninsured American might pay 20 to 100 percent more for a drug than large American insurance plans pay. Some countries bargain aggressively for lower drug prices and provide subsidies to ensure that those who need to use the drugs will purchase them. The average retail price for a month's supply of Lipitor, for example, which does a great job at lowering cholesterol levels, is $68 in the United States, $48 in Canada, $34 in the United Kingdom, and less

than $30 in Germany. My $34 bottle of nasal steroid (for sinusitis) broke somewhere over the Atlantic, between Baltimore and Annecy, France. I was astonished when the local French pharmacy replaced it for $3.50. The pharmaceutical industry rightly argues that it needs to recoup the expense of discovering new drugs, but Americans might legitimately ask why they pay most of the costs for new drugs that benefit Canadians, Germans, and the British. Besides, large pharmaceutical firms spend ten times more on marketing than on research.

* Physicians need to be given incentives to choose specialties (such as primary care) and locations (inner cities and rural areas) that desperately need them. These specialties and practice locations generally pay poorly and demand long and unpredictable working hours. As care becomes more complex, it has become more fragmented. If Americans are to receive coordinated care as whole patients—and not just for their disease du jour—someone must see to that. If not a physician, then someone trained in everything needed to coordinate care without being a physician.

* "Evidence-based medicine" needs to become the norm. (I've always thought the average American would be startled to learn that we physicians hadn't been so attentive to proven "evidence" in the past.) Professional societies have begun to develop clinical practice guidelines, which make clear, from the best evidence available, what works (and what doesn't) and at what cost. Because patients differ, one size will never fit all, but on average, similar patients with similar conditions require roughly similar care. Excluding ineffective and unproven interventions improves care and lowers costs.

No one claims that implementing a new, transparent, rational system that addresses these critical issues will be easy, but it would be an enormous improvement.

In the absence of federal action, states have begun to enact newer, more inclusive systems. While not yet "universal," these recognize the need to provide relief to small businesses and the self-employed and ultimately strive for cost-efficient and effective ways to provide good-quality care to the poor. But individual states do not have the depth and breadth of resources and controls that the federal government can deploy. In 2008, Oregon's 600,000 uninsured vied, by lottery, for 24,000 state-financed health insurance policies.

Change may be in the wind. The 2008 national elections resulted in a seismic shift in the U.S. political landscape. The Democrats, who have long favored significant expansion of health care coverage and meaningful reform, strengthened their control of both houses of Congress and took the White House. Universal coverage has often emerged in nations at moments of societal crisis, whether the Great Depression or World War II. Neither worked for the United States: Roosevelt was forced to strike it from his 1935 New Deal legislation, and Truman had to abandon its passage following World War II.

This time might be different. Meaningful reform will gore more than the occasional ox. The growth in health care spending requires that efficiencies and savings must be wrung from any new "system." We must eliminate the inefficiencies of the health insurance sector, the outsized profits of "big pharma," and the abiding insistence of many Americans that they receive all the care the want—whenever they want it.

Fifteen years ago, J. H. Brody summed up the attributes of U.S. health care: "the current system provides appropriate high-quality care to a small group, inappropriately complex care to a larger group, and virtually no care at all to far too many."[9] Since then, things have only gotten worse. One powerful impetus for change is a growing recognition and resentment of America's health disparities.

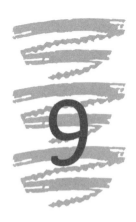

Who's Healthy?
Who's Not? Why?

"Health disparities" is the new rallying cry among those concerned about social equality. I'm not talking about the great divide between people living in wealthy, stable nations and those living in countries that are poor and politically turbulent. I'm talking about systematic differences in the health of Americans.

For whatever reasons (and there are many), Americans experience vastly different states of "health." White women have the longest life expectancy; black men have the shortest. On average, black men die six years earlier than white men (1.4 of those lost years are attributable to heart disease; another year, to homicides). Black men who live in Harlem (and places like Harlem) have the shortest life expectancy of all; shorter, in fact, than the citizens of Bangladesh (Figure 29). If black Americans were a nation, their life expectancy would be shorter than that of the populations of 104 other countries.

Some of this has to do with larger social and economic forces (drug use, gun violence, low literacy rates, unemployment, single-

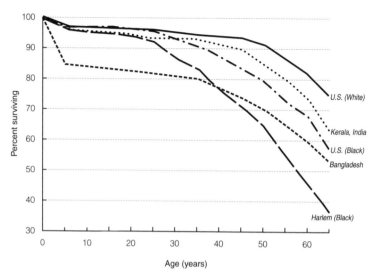

FIGURE 29. SEEING IS BELIEVING.
Survival rates for males in selected demographics. Black men in America have died at much younger ages, on average, than white men. Black men in Harlem have died at much younger ages than male Indians in the state of Kerala or, after about age 45, male Bangladeshis. Source: Reprinted with permission from A. Sen, "The Economics of Life and Death," *Scientific American* (May 1993), 45. Copyright © 1993 Scientific American, Inc. All rights reserved.

parent households, racism). But some of it doesn't. Some of the causes are so intertwined that they are difficult to sort out.

Some determinants are no doubt "genetic." But, even then, it is not always clear which factor is nurture and which is nature: the influences of a group's DNA or of its shared behavior and environment.

On average, black women have the highest rates of obesity of any major ethnic group in the United States. Is that because they are genetically prone to a different body habitus than white women (calorie for calorie, more is retained) or because they consume more calories and exercise less (which is important for better health, though less so for weight)? There is probably no single answer, but exactly where one's ancestors came from probably affects one's body type. Some Africans are the tallest, leanest, and swiftest humans on Earth, but not all, and not the average African American. Genes have an influence, however slight and however complex. So do culture and behavior.

Different cultures have different dietary preferences. Soon after I became dean of the Bloomberg School of Public Health, we received a foundation grant to work closely with the communities with which we share our East Baltimore location. Many of the community leaders were local pastors, with whom I'd meet once every month or two, often over dinner, to discuss progress. Dinner meetings alternated between the school and one of the pastor's churches. Whenever we met at the school, I would provide a buffet spread of grilled chicken, salad, vegetables, breads, and dessert. Some months later, one of my pastor colleagues let me in on a secret: after "dinner meetings" held at the school, the pastors would all go out to eat. Grilled chicken, salad, and vegetables were not considered "dinner"; fried chicken would have been a start![1]

A study published in the *New England Journal of Medicine* recorded the exercise patterns of school-aged girls (exercise was defined in the broadest sense). Among both white and black adolescents, metabolic expenditure on exercise declines rapidly with age, but it declines much more among black girls (Figure 30).

Some differences aren't understood at all. African Americans are far more prone to high blood pressure than are whites. High blood pressure tends to be familial (i.e., it probably has some genetic basis, as complex and diluted as that might be). Ditto the fact that blacks are four times more likely to develop blinding glaucoma.

African American women are also more likely to give birth to low-

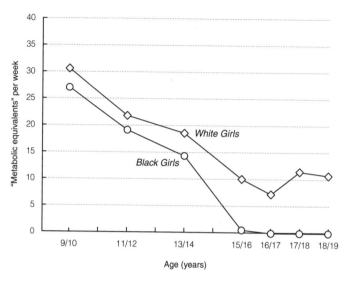

Daily Physical Activity of Schoolgirls
United States

FIGURE 30. EXERCISE SEEMS TO BE FOR THE VERY YOUNG.
Daily physical activity of schoolgirls ages 9 through 19 in the United States. "Metabolic equivalents" of activity declined rapidly as adolescents aged—more dramatically among black girls. *Source: Reprinted with permission from S. Kim, N. W. Glynn, A. M. Kriska, et al., "Decline in Physical Activity in Black Girls and White Girls during Adolescence," New England Journal of Medicine 347 (2002): 713, Figure 2. Copyright © 2002 Massachusetts Medical Society. All rights reserved.*

birth-weight offspring—well-educated, well-off, professional black women. Clearly, something more than wealth, education, good nutrition, and prenatal care is at work.

If we can't remove innate risks, we could, through more effective health care programs, minimize their impact. Screening blacks earlier and more frequently for hypertension and glaucoma would allow earlier detection and therapy, reducing complications (heart attack and stroke in the case of hypertension, blindness in the case of glaucoma).

There is little doubt that poverty, ignorance, and discrimination combine in powerful and complex ways that adversely affect health.

These societal factors are difficult to deal with. The poor often eat poorly because they have little choice: more nutritious diets (fish, fresh salad, and vegetables) cost more and often aren't available to inner-city communities. Liquor stores and liquor ads target poor neighborhoods, and tobacco companies concoct mentholated brands that appeal to the tastes of inner-city black youth. There are few local opportunities for employment, forcing the inner-city poor to travel great distances, often by inadequate public transport, to get to jobs. The poor are often unable to obtain health insurance (their employers don't offer benefits, and insurance companies consider them high risk). Health care, when available, often comes from overwhelmed public or charitable clinics. Mothers have told me that having a child immunized fills a day: report to one office (where they may wait hours) for the necessary permits, then travel across town by inefficient public transport to get the shots. Single mothers are frequently forced to choose between a day's meager but critical wage and having a child immunized. Sometimes, losing a few days of work to tend to a sick child can cost a mother her job. Hence the overuse of emergency rooms.

The health consequences of Michael Marmot's "social gradient of disease" (Chapter 4), in which those receiving orders are less healthy than those doing the ordering, is a subtle, if powerful, contributor to U.S. health disparities. So are subtly (if unintentionally) "biased" physicians. Black men and women presenting with symptoms of heart disease are less likely to be referred for expensive tests and interventions, even by black physicians, than are their white counterparts.

In rare instances, innovative health care tools have countered disparities whose origins were never clear in the first place. Historically, black children were far more likely than white children to have bouts of bacterial pneumonia. By 2002, this difference had largely disappeared (Figure 31). What had occurred during the interim? An

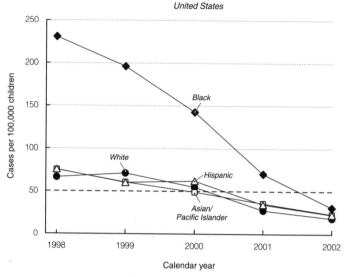

Incidence of Invasive Pneumococcal Disease among Children Younger than 5 Years

United States

FIGURE 31. NEW TOOLS CAN MITIGATE HEALTH DISPARITIES.
Incidence of invasive pneumococcal disease among children younger than five years in the United States. The introduction of routine immunization of American children with a newly developed conjugate pneumococcal vaccine reduced serious infections in all racial groups, especially blacks, virtually eliminating what had been a longstanding health disparity between black and white youth. Source: Reprinted with permission from B. Flannery, S. Schrag, and N. M. Bennett, "Impact of Childhood Vaccination on Racial Disparities in Invasive Streptococcus pneumoniae Infections," Journal of the American Medical Association 291 (2004): 2199, Figure 1. Copyright © 2004 American Medical Association. All rights reserved.

effective pneumococcal vaccine was developed and deployed for all young children.

As we focus more attention on the causes of and solutions to health disparities, the gaps should narrow. But this improvement will take sustained commitment of time and resources. The same could be said for the health of all Americans: it will improve as Americans adopt healthier lifestyles and as better, more cost-effective interventions are developed and made available to all.

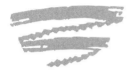

Notes

Chapter 1. Genesis

1. The first major outbreak of plague followed the return of Genovese merchant ships to Sicily from the plague-wracked Crimea in October 1347. By 1351, Florence's population had been cut in half. In parts of Italy, France, and Spain, 75 percent of the population perished. The pestilence returned repeatedly over the next couple of centuries, more or less disappearing as a serious health threat when transmission declined. For the most part unknowingly, humans erected more effective barriers between themselves and disease-carrying rats: houses were sturdier structures; the gray, ground-burrowing rat replaced the brown house rat as the dominant species; and better sanitation, quarantine, and other public health measures were deployed more widely and effectively. Few modern depictions of the cultural dislocation and abject fear generated by the fourteenth-century plagues match Ingmar Bergman's classic film from 1957, The Seventh Seal.

2. C. P. Snow, The Two Cultures (Cambridge: Cambridge University Press, 1998), 83.

3. Rousseau, quoted in W. H. Foege, "In search of a national agenda for international health problems," American Journal of Tropical Medicine and Hygiene 42 (1990): 293–97.

4. J. B. McKinlay and S. M. McKinlay, "The questionable contribution of medical measures to the decline of mortality in the United States in the twentieth century," *Milbank Memorial Fund Quarterly: Health and Society* 55 (1977): 405–28.

Chapter 2. Disease Is the Sum of All Evils

1. Even "ordinary" tuberculosis now requires long treatment with multiple antibiotics to ensure a cure. Unfortunately, patients feel much improved long before their six- to nine-month course of treatment is completed. Every time a patient fails to complete the treatment because he or she is feeling better, the few remaining, hardy tubercle bacilli receive a reprieve—and all too frequently re-emerge, months to years later, resistant to everything in our antibiotic arsenal.

2. The strategy on which the entire global eradication effort had originally been based was to vaccinate everyone. Unfortunately, public health programs never reach everyone. A sample survey of the population of Delhi, conducted before the initiation of a program meant to vaccinate everyone in the city, indicated that 85 percent of the population displayed the residual scars of prior vaccination. After the intensive campaign reportedly vaccinated more than 100 percent of Delhi's population, the prevalence of vaccination scars remained unchanged, at 85 percent! One can never come face to face with much more than 85 percent of a population, whether for a health intervention or for an electoral campaign.

3. More than 90 percent of U.S. children receive their recommended immunizations. But those who don't, often clustered in communities of doubters, risk becoming infected (often by an unimmunized individual returning from overseas). A local outbreak then threatens the lives of those too young or too immunologically compromised by illness to be vaccinated. Parents who refuse immunizations exemplify the inequitable nature of the "tragedy of the commons." They withhold immunization from their children to preclude the rare possibility of vaccine-related complications, trusting that immunization of other parents' children will protect theirs from the spread of disease—a perceived personal gain at the expense of the public's good, except their child remains at risk! During 2008, the United States experienced more mea-

sles cases than during any year in recent memory; unimmunized children were twenty times as likely to become ill as those who had received their measles "shots."

4. Drs. Luc Montagnier and Françoise Barré-Sinoussi received the 2008 Nobel Prize for having discovered the HIV virus in 1983.

5. What we can predict is that new influenza viruses will constantly emerge. During April and May of 2009, as page proofs for this book were being assembled, a novel ("swine") influenza A (H1N1) virus emerged in the Americas and quickly circled the globe. It also stole the headlines from avian (H5N1) influenza. While the novel influenza (H1N1) virus is far more contagious than avian (H5N1) virus, so far it is (thankfully) much less lethal. It also remains sensitive to Tamiflu. But seasonal H1N1 was also sensitive during the 2007–2008 flu season but now is almost entirely resistant.

6. Dr. Harald zur Hausen, of Heidelberg, Germany, received the 2008 Nobel Prize for having discovered that human papilloma virus was responsible for cervical cancer and that some strains were much more oncogenic than others.

CHAPTER 3. GENES

1. Ludwig J. J. Wittgenstein, Philosophical Investigations (Cambridge, MA: Blackwell Publishers, 1958), 212.

CHAPTER 4. THE COMPLEX NATURE OF CAUSALITY

1. Matt Ridley, Genome: The Autobiography of a Species in 23 Chapters (New York: HarperCollins, 1999).

CHAPTER 5. THE CONSEQUENCES OF OUR OWN BEHAVIOR

1. Compounding the difficulties inherent in getting lifelong smokers to quit—habit, clan culture, and nicotine addiction—is the newly discovered fact that smokers with a particular genetic variation are likely to light up more cigarettes each day than are those without it. They are also more likely to develop lung cancer.

2. By 2007, only 8.5 percent of New York high school students smoked (down from 17.6 percent in 2001), compared with 23 percent of high school students nationwide (2005 data).

3. "Overweight" is clinically defined as a body mass index (BMI) of 25 or above; "obese" as a BMI of 30 or above. Someone 5 feet 6 inches tall would be "overweight" at 155 pounds and "obese" at 186 pounds. Someone 6 feet tall would be "overweight" at 184 pounds and "obese" at 221 pounds. A recent survey suggests that the obesity epidemic among U.S. children may have peaked. Only time will tell. In any case, rates are already far too high for our collective good.

4. As Michael Pollan advises in his recent book, In Defense of Food (New York: Penguin, 2008), "Eat food [meaning 'something your grandmother would have recognized' as food]. Not too much. Mostly plants."

5. Steven Jones, "Genetics in medicine: Real promises, unreal expectations. One scientist's advice to policymakers in the United Kingdom and the United States," Milbank Memorial Fund, New York, New York, June 2008.

6. Those societal webs that encourage and spread unhealthy behavior can work in reverse. A recent study found that people generally stop smoking not individually but in closely connected groups. One author likened it to observing celestial events: "It's not like one little star turning off at a time . . . Whole constellations are blinking off at once."

CHAPTER 6. CHOOSING THE HEALTHIER LIFESTYLE

1. New York Times, March 22, 1998.

2. Baltimore Sun, July 25, 1994.

3. New York Times, December 18, 2007.

4. A vocal minority strongly believes that vaccines cause autism; most are parents and relatives of autistic children. Because autism commonly makes its appearance during the second year of life, when children receive many of their "shots," most instances of autism are first noticed by parents within weeks or months of an immunization. Despite the lack of any credible evidence, their views, and those of other advocates who believe vaccines are responsible for other disorders as well, have raised general concerns among the public. Some surveys have found that 80 percent of U.S. parents now harbor concerns about recommended childhood immunizations, though the vast majority ultimately heed the advice of their pediatricians and have their children immunized.

Chapter 7. From Science to Policy

1. It's hard to prove a negative, particularly when it is a moving target. The aforementioned antivaccine autism advocates are a telling case in point. Recently, a socially prominent, long-time supporter of medical research asked me to design a study that would settle, once and for all, the "debate" about the purported role of vaccines in the development of autism. I almost rose to the bait. I soon learned that no study would ever satisfy the concerns of the advocates: they had a long history of changing the nature of their concern. Their original villain was the combined measles-mumps-rubella vaccine. When studies demonstrated that this was not the culprit, a vaccine preservative, mercury-based thimerasol, was blamed. When thimerasol was removed from most vaccines and the rate of autism continued unabated, the culprit became the schedule with which vaccines are administered. It is hard enough to prove that x doesn't cause y. It is virtually impossible when the purported x keeps changing!

Chapter 8. The U.S. Health Care System

1. A recent study detected a genetic variation that explains, in part, why some patients with heart failure respond to a class of drugs (beta blockers) while others don't. Particularly important, from a public health perspective, is that the variation is present in only 2 percent of white Americans but 40 percent of black Americans. Should these early results prove correct, the very high frequency in blacks might make screening for this genetic marker useful, as it could save large numbers of patients the cost and risk of complications associated with a drug from which they can't possibly benefit.

2. While the populations of very poor countries invariably have short life expectancy, the causes that underlie international differences in life expectancy are complicated by differences in the social, cultural, and physical environments in which people live, wide disparities in expenditures on health services for the elite versus the masses (which can distort metrics such as "mean expenditure"), and poorly quantified investments in critical public health measures. For example, South Africa spends $437 per capita on health care, nearly 100 times the $6 spent by

Ethiopia. But life expectancy is reportedly five years longer in Ethiopia than it is in South Africa (56 versus 51 years).

3. D. F. Stroup and S. M. Teutsch (editors), *Statistics in Public Health: Quantitative Approaches to Public Health Problems* (New York: Oxford University Press, 1998), 4.

4. Roy Porter, *The Greatest Benefit to Mankind: A Medical History of Humanity* (New York: Norton, 1997).

5. Other "market force" organizations have found ways to profit from "managing" my care. My employer, the Johns Hopkins University, decided that one way to reduce its costs for my medical benefits is to turn my insured drug coverage over to a large pharmaceutical management firm. How does this reduce costs? In part, by making it more difficult for me to obtain my drugs! The management company's most economical purchasing plan requires me to buy three months worth of whatever drug I need and prohibits me from ordering a refill until the three months are up. Because I travel internationally for long periods, the refill date frequently coincides with my being overseas. When I called to refill a prescription one week ahead of time, so as to have the medicine I would need for the four weeks I would be out of the country, I was told by two "customer representatives" that it would be impossible for me to obtain my drugs ahead of time. After wasting more than an hour at the Website of the management company and on additional fruitless phone calls, I finally reached someone who said, "This is not a problem. We will simply provide you with a special 'vacation authorization.' But you can get this only once a year." My problem, of course, was that it was not a vacation, and I would fall into this trap more than once a year. I heard the same complaint, about this same "catch-22," from an irate listener on National Public Radio. This piling on of bureaucratic rules and procedures may improve the management company's (and Johns Hopkins's) bottom line, but it does nothing to improve patients' compliance with their prescribed medical therapies. My secretary, who is covered by the same plan and makes a good deal less in salary than I do, long ago abandoned the three-monthly mailings and instead buys her medicines one month at a time at the local drug store—our most expensive but ultimately most convenient option.

6. J. M. McWilliams, E. Meara, A. M. Zaslovsky, and J. Z. Ayanian,

"Health of previously uninsured adults after acquiring Medicare coverage," JAMA 298 (2007): 2886–94.

7. Interestingly, within one year of enacting its local attempt at universal health insurance, the proportion of uninsured in the state of Massachusetts declined by half, regardless of income level.

8. Employer Health Benefits, 2008 Annual Survey, The Kaiser Family Foundation and Health Research and Educational Trust, http://ehbs.kff .org/pdf/, accessed December 10, 2008.

9. H. Brody, H. V. Sparks, W. S. Abbett, D. L. Wood, W. C. Wodland, and R. C. Smith, "The mammalian medical center for the twenty-first century," JAMA 270 (1993): 1097–1100.

CHAPTER 9. WHO'S HEALTHY? WHO'S NOT? WHY?

1. The reasons for disparities in health between white and black Americans can be both subtle and complex. In a recent study of individual physicians treating both black and white patients with diabetes, blacks were tested as often but were less successful in controlling their diabetes—even when their physicians were providing high-quality care. The authors concluded that the problem might lie, in part, in the physician's providing the same counseling and care to patients whose cultural milieus varied widely—perhaps preferring either deep-fried to grilled chicken as a culturally appropriate (and socially enforced) cultural norm.

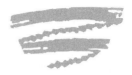

Further Reading, Films,
and Websites of Interest

The number of books, journal articles, movies, and Websites relevant to the subjects I've discussed is virtually limitless. For those with the time and interest, I list here a few of my favorites. They add considerable depth and color to this book's summary of core principles. Included are some helpful and largely reliable Websites for up-to-date information and recommendations.

Life before Modern Public Health
Bergman, Ingmar (director). The Seventh Seal. Criterion, 1956, film.
McNeill, William H. Plagues and Peoples. New York: Doubleday, 1977.
Tuchman, Barbara W. A Distant Mirror: The Calamitous Fourteenth Century. New York: Random House, 1978.

The Discovery of Microbes: A Classic Tale
De Kruif, Paul. Microbe Hunters. New York: Harcourt, 1926.

The Effects of Infectious Disease on Society
Mann, Thomas. The Magic Mountain. Translation by John E. Woods. New York: Vintage, 1996.

Rothman, Sheila M. *Living in the Shadow of Death: Tuberculosis and the Social Experience of Illness in American History.* New York: Harper-Collins, 1995.

Zinsser, Hans. *Rats, Lice, and History.* Boston: Little, Brown, 1934.

BATTLING INFECTIOUS DISEASE

Barry, John M. *The Great Influenza: The Epic Story of the Deadliest Plague in History.* New York: Penguin, 2004.

Davies, Peter. *The Devil's Flu.* New York: Henry Holt, 1959.

Fenner, F., D. A. Henderson, I. Arita, Z. Jezek, and I. D. Ladnyi. *Smallpox and Its Eradication.* Geneva: World Health Organization, 1988.

Garrett, Laurie. *Betrayal of Trust: The Collapse of Global Public Health.* New York: Hyperion, 2000.

Oshinsky, David M. *Polio: An American Story.* New York: Oxford University Press, 2005.

Packard, Randall M. *The Making of a Tropical Disease: A Short History of Malaria.* Baltimore: Johns Hopkins University Press, 2007.

Ryan, Frank. *The Forgotten Plague: How the Battle against Tuberculosis Was Won—and Lost.* Boston: Little, Brown, 1992.

NONINFECTIOUS DISEASE, EPIDEMIOLOGY, AND THE NATURE OF EVIDENCE

Brandt, Allan M. *The Cigarette Century: The Rise, Fall, and Deadly Persistence of the Product That Defined America.* New York: Basic Books, 2007.

Huber, Peter W. *Galileo's Revenge: Junk Science in the Courtroom.* New York: Basic Books, 1991.

Mann, Michael (director). *The Insider.* Buena Vista Pictures, 1999, film.

Marmot, Michael, and Richard G. Wilkinson. *Social Determinants of Health.* Oxford: Oxford University Press, 1999.

Pollan, Michael. *In Defense of Food: An Eater's Manifesto.* New York: Penguin, 2008.

Ridley, Matt. *Genome: The Autobiography of a Species in 23 Chapters.* New York: HarperCollins, 1999.

Schlosser, Eric. *Fast Food Nation: The Dark Side of the All-American Meal.* New York: Houghton Mifflin, 2001

U.S. Department of Health and Human Services. *The Health Conse-*

quences of Involuntary Exposure to Tobacco Smoke: A Report of the Surgeon General. U.S. Department of Health and Human Services, Centers for Disease Control and Prevention, Coordinating Center for Health Promotion, National Center for Chronic Disease Prevention and Health Promotion, Office on Smoking and Health, 2006. (All Surgeon General's Reports on Smoking are also available online: www.cdc.gov/tobacco.)

U.S. Department of Health, Education, and Welfare. Smoking and Health: Report of the Advisory Committee to the Surgeon General of the Public Health Service. Washington, D.C.: U.S. Public Health Service. Office of the Surgeon General, 1964.

Woodham-Smith, Cecil. The Great Hunger: Ireland, 1845–1849. London: Penguin, 1962

MEDICAL CARE, POLICY, AND OUTCOMES

Brownlee, Shannon. Overtreated: Why Too Much Medicine Is Making Us Sicker and Poorer. New York: Bloomsbury USA, 2008.

Porter, Roy. The Greatest Benefit to Mankind: A Medical History of Humanity. New York: Norton, 1997.

INFORMATIONAL WEBSITES

American Cancer Society: www.cancer.org

American Heart Association: www.americanheart.org

Centers for Disease Control and Prevention: www.cdc.gov

Clinical Practice Guidelines: www.guideline.gov

Commonwealth Fund: www.commonwealthfund.org

Dartmouth Atlas of Health Care: www.dartmouthatlas.org

Healthy People 2010: www.healthypeople.gov

Institute for Vaccine Safety: www.vaccinesafety.edu

Institute of Medicine: www.iom.edu

Kaiser Family Foundation: www.kff.org

National Institutes of Health: www.nih.gov

Organization for Economic Cooperation and Development: www.oecd.org/health

Preventive Services Task Force: www.ahrq.gov/clinic/prevnew.htm

World Health Organization: www.who.int/en

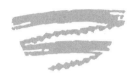

Index

Bernie, Leroy, 42
Berry, Donald, 72
beta blockers, 119n1 (chap. 8)
beta-carotene, 58, 60
bifurcated needles, 14, 15
bird flu. *See* avian influenza
birth control pills, 72
Black Death, 2, 12, 115n1
Bloomberg, Michael R., 43–44, 45
Blue Cross / Blue Shield, 75, 94–95
Botox injections, 96
breast cancer: death rates from, 38–39, 40; and genetic risk factors, 29; screening for, 71–72, 100
Brody, J. H., 107–8
bronchitis, 40
Brownell, Kelly, 36, 53
bypass surgery, 89, 90

calcium, 61
Canada, health care system in, 88–89
cancer: cervical, 23–25; colon, 59, 96; death rates for men, 41; death rates for women, 39–40; infection as factor in, 22–25; liver, 23, 35; stomach, 23, 27. *See also* breast cancer; lung cancer
capitation, 84–85, 86
cardiovascular disease: and smoking, 40; stroke's risk factors, 31. *See also* heart disease
cataract surgery, 85, 86
causality, complexity of, 32–36, 57–58

Centers for Disease Control and Prevention (CDC), 45, 65
Centers for Healthcare Research and Quality, 88
Cerezyme, 96
cervical cancer, 23–25
cesarean section, 86–88
children: diseases in, 6, 11; and obesity, 36, 45; and risks from cold medicines, 69
China, population fluctuations in, 2–3
chondroitin sulfate, 60–61
clinical guidelines, 83–84, 106
Coca-Cola, 36
colon cancer, 59, 96
co-payments, as factor in health care delivery, 100
cortisol, 33
cowpox, 14
Creutzfeldt-Jakob disease, 22–23
C-section, 86–88

death: in early childhood, 4, 5; median age of, 4, 5. *See also* life expectancy
dermatologists, 96
diabetes, 31, 49, 51, 121n1
diarrhea, 11
Dickens, Charles, 35
diet and nutrition, 118n4 (chap. 5); cultural differences in, 111, 121n1; as factor in health and illness, 27, 45–52; fads in, 64
diphtheria, 11
disease: causes of, 10–11, 32–36;

fetal origins of, 35–36; infectious, 11–13; prevention of, 85; racial variations in risk of, 29, 30. *See also specific diseases*

doctors. *See physicians*

Doll, Richard, 42

drugs: competitive pricing for, 105–6; insurance coverage for, 120n5. *See also pharmaceutical companies*

early childhood diseases, 6, 11

Eaton, Bill, 32

emergency rooms, 99–100

emphysema, 40, 41

endocrine disrupters, 35

England, health care rationing in, 89–92

environment, as risk factor, 34–36. *See also living conditions*

evidence-based medicine, 67–72, 106

exercise, 112

experience rating, 95

family planning, 6

Farr, William, 84

Fertility Diet, 62–63

fertility rates, 6

fetal monitoring, 86–88

fiber, 59

finasteride, 68

folic acid, 59

Food and Drug Administration, 65, 68

Frenk, Julio, 10

Frieden, Tom, 43, 53

Frist, Bill, 72

gastritis, 23

Gates, Bill, 45

Gaucher disease, 96

Genentech, 96–97

genes, as factor in health and disease, 26–31, 110

genetic screening, 29–30

Genzyme, 96

germs. *See infection; microbes*

glaucoma, 30, 85, 111, 112

hair loss, 68

Hausen, Harald zur, 117n6

health: diet as factor in, 27; educating the public about, 52–53; genes as factor in, 26–31; living conditions as factor in, 6–9; obesity as factor in, 45–52; smoking as factor in, 27–29, 83–45; social and economic factors affecting, 109–10, 112–13, 119–20n2; social status as factor in, 33–34, 113

health care: in Canada, 88–89, 102; co-payments as factor in, 100; disparities in, 80, 108, 109–14, 121n1; measuring quality of, 77–79; overall benefits of providing, 101–3; as a public good, 101; rationing of, 89–92; in the United Kingdom, 89–92; universal, 79, 100–103, 107. *See also public health*

health care costs (U.S.), 89, 101–2; and clinical practice guidelines, 83–84, 106; for clinical trials, 88; in comparison with other countries, 76–78; and co-payments, 100; for drugs, 105–6; growth of, 77, 78, 103; hidden, 101–2; and market forces, 92–100, 120n5; for Medicare, 82–83, 84; public financing of, 101–2; reducing, 102; technology as factor in, 85–88; variations in, 79–80, 82–84

health care professionals. See nurses; physicians

health care system, U.S.: coordination of patient care under, 74, 106; dissatisfaction with, 97–98; practice guidelines for, 83–84, 106; problems inherent in, 73–75; reform of, 104–8. See also public health

health claims: by medical researchers, 55–63; by the pharmaceutical industry, 63–65; as reported in the media, 54–55, 65; scientific evidence for, 67–72, 106; validity of, 65–66

health insurance plans, 75, 100–101; comparison shopping for, 105; difficulty of choosing, 94–96; as employee benefit, 75, 94–96; and health screenings, 85; state plans, 107, 121n7; supplemental, 105

health maintenance organizations (HMOs), 85

health outcomes. See health; life expectancy

heart attack: aspirin for, 67; surgical intervention after, 89, 90

heart disease: death rates from, 37–38, 39; and genetic factors, 119n1 (chap. 8); risk factors for, 27, 31

Helicobacter pylori, 13, 23

hepatitis, 23

high blood pressure, 31; among African Americans, 111, 112

Hippocrates, 6–7

HIV/AIDS, 13, 15, 20–21, 117n4; and needle-exchange programs, 71; risk factors for, 31; transmission of, 21, 71

homocysteine, 59

hormone replacement therapy (HRT), 61–62

human papilloma virus (HPV), 13; and cervical cancer, 23–25, 117n6

Huntington disease, 30

Hutchison, Kay Bailey, 72

hypertension, 31; among African Americans, 111, 112

immunization, 113, 116–17n3. See also vaccines

infant mortality rates, 5, 78–79

infection, 11–13; as factor in cancer, 22–25; spread of, 8–9; and stress, 33

influenza: avian, 12, 22, 117n5; forecasts for outbreaks of, 22; H1N1 (swine), 117n5
infomercials, 64–65
Institute of Medicine, 66
insurance companies, profitability of, 93–94. *See also* health insurance plans
interleukin 2, 33

James, King, 41
Japan, health policy in, 72
Jenner, Edward, 14
Jews, and risk of Tay-Sachs disease, 29
Jones, Steve, 51
Juvenile Diabetes Association, 66

Kaiser, Henry, 75
Kaiser-Permanente, 85

Lamm, Richard, 80
Lee, J. W., 22
life expectancy, 3–9; demographic group differences in, 109–14, 119–20n2; increases in, 6; and living conditions, 6–9; as measure of health care quality, 78–79; U.S., as compared with other countries, 78–79
liver cancer, 23, 35
living conditions, as factor in life expectancy, 6–9, 31
Lucentis, 97
lung cancer: epidemiology of, 27–28; in men, 41; and smoking,

27–29, 39–42, 117n1 (chap. 5); in women, 39–40

mad cow disease, 22–23
mammography, 71–72
Marmot, Michael, 33–34, 113
Marshall, Barry, 23
maternal death, 11
McKinlay, J. B., 9
McKinlay, S. M., 9
measles, 11, 116–17n3; deaths from, 6, 7, 12
Medicaid, 75, 98–99, 101, 103, 104–5
medical practice: under capitation, 84–85; variations in, 79–80, 83–84, 85–88, 89
medical research: assessing validity of, 64–66; confusion regarding, 54–64; and health policy, 67–72, 106; reliability of, 54–56, 65–66
medical technology, as factor in health care spending, 85–88
Medicare, 75, 98, 101, 102, 103; costs of, 82–83, 84
methicillin-resistant *Staphylococcus aureus* (MRSA), 13
microbes: as cause of cancer, 22–25; evolution of, 11–13
Montagnier, Luc, 117n4
Moynihan, Patrick, 82
multivitamins, 59

National Cancer Institute (NCI), 71–72

ALFRED SOMMER is an internationally recognized medical researcher, educator, and administrator who has spent his career seeking better ways to prevent and treat disease. He received his medical education at Harvard and his training in ophthalmology and epidemiology at Johns Hopkins, where he is now a professor of ophthalmology, epidemiology, and international health. He is best known globally for his pioneering discovery that inexpensive vitamin A supplements can save the lives of a million young children every year, a finding that the World Bank, among other institutions, has judged to be one of the most cost-effective of all medical interventions. Among ophthalmologists, he is recognized for spearheading blindness-prevention programs and for initiating the development of clinical treatment guidelines by the American Academy of Ophthalmology.

Sommer was dean of the Johns Hopkins Bloomberg School of Public Health from 1990 to 2005. He has published more than 250 scientific articles and 5 books and has received numerous awards, including the Albert Lasker Clinical Medical Research Award. He is an elected member of both the Institute of Medicine and the National Academy of Sciences.